WITHDRAWN

TOUCH IN PSYCHOTHERAPY

THEORY IN PSYCHOTHERAPY

TOUCH IN PSYCHOTHERAPY

THEORY, RESEARCH, AND PRACTICE

Edited by

**Edward W. L. Smith
Pauline Rose Clance
Suzanne Imes**

THE GUILFORD PRESS
New York   London

© 1998 The Guilford Press
A Division of Guilford Publications, Inc.
72 Spring Street, New York, NY 10012
http://www.guilford.com

All rights reserved

No part of this book may be reproduced, stored in a retrieval system, or transmitted, in any form or by any means, electronic, mechanical, photocopying, microfilming, recording, or otherwise, without written permission from the Publisher.

Printed in the United States of America

This book is printed on acid-free paper.

Last digit is print number: 9 8 7 6 5 4 3 2 1

Library of Congress Cataloging-in-Publication Data

Touch in psychotherapy : theory, research, and practice /
    Edward W. L. Smith, Pauline Rose Clance, Suzanne Imes, editors.
        p. cm.
    Includes bibliographical references and index.
    ISBN 1-57230-269-0 (hard)
    1. Touch—Therapeutic use. 2. Psychotherapy. 3. Touch—
Psychological aspects. I. Smith, Edward W. L., 1942–
II. Clance, Pauline Rose. III. Imes, Suzanne.
RC489.T69T68 1998
616'89'14—dc21   97-41416
                                                             CIP

CONTRIBUTORS

Reuven Bar-Levav, MD, is a psychiatrist who practices and teaches a basically new form of intensive individual and group psychotherapy in Southfield, Michigan, just outside Detroit. He and his group do not address the cerebral cortex, but aim at changing the physiological adjustments that formed early in life; this can undercut the anxiety and reverse lifelong depression. Process always comes before content. His approach is based on the realization that thinking, insight, understanding, and interpretations are all relatively powerless vis-à-vis raw emotions, before they have been experienced and fully expressed in very safe settings, where acting out is strictly forbidden. Dr. Bar-Levav is a widely published writer, a contributing editor of *Voices,* an ex-editor of *The Detroit Medical News,* and the author of *Thinking in the Shadow of Feelings: A New Understanding of the Hidden Forces That Shape Individuals and Societies* (Simon & Schuster, 1988). His latest best-selling book, *Every Family Needs a C.E.O.: What Mothers and Fathers Can Do About Our Deteriorating Families and Values,* was published in 1995 by Fathering.

Susan Chance, MS, is a PhD student in the Department of Psychology at Georgia State University in Atlanta, where she received her bachelor's and master's degrees. She has done a great deal of work in the area of understanding and preventing suicide. Her other areas of interest are psychotherapy (particularly long-term psychodynamic treatment); object relations theories and their application to the psychotherapeutic process; supervision; and developmental psychology. She has several publications in the areas of psychotherapy, object relations theory, and the understanding of suicide.

Pauline Rose Clance, PhD, ABPP, is a professor of psychology at Georgia State University and is a former chair of the GSU Clinical Psychology Program. She teaches advanced psychotherapy courses at GSU and is a clinical supervisor for students who are seeing clients in the GSU Psychology Clinic. She is an associate editor of the *Gestalt Review* and is on the editorial board of *Psychotherapy: Theory, Research, and Practice* and the *Journal of Couples Therapy*. She has a private practice and works with individuals, couples, and groups. She has received a diploma in clinical psychology from the American Board of Professional Psychology (ABPP).

Joen Fagan, PhD, ABPP, before retiring, served on the graduate faculty at Georgia State University for 30 years, holding the position of Regents' Professor of Psychology. She specialized in psychotherapy training, holistic approaches to healing, and dissociative disorders. Her best-known publications are *Gestalt Therapy Now* (coedited with Irma Lee Shepherd; Science and Behavior Books, 1970) and *Incipient Multiple Personality in Childhood* (coauthored with Polly Paul McMahan).

Pamela Geib, EdD, is an instructor in psychology in the Department of Psychiatry at Harvard Medical School. She is on the faculty of the Couples and Family Training Program at the Cambridge Hospital, and maintains private practices in Cambridge and Newton, Massachusetts. Her areas of interest include working with individuals and families who are struggling with physical limitations; the intersection of spiritual and psychological domains in psychotherapy; and treatment of couples in which one member is a trauma survivor. She has contributed chapters to the books *On Intimate Ground: A Gestalt Approach to Working with Couples,* and *The Voice of Shame: Silence and Connection in Psychotherapy.* She has also coauthored the paper "Consciousness of Context in Relational Couples Therapy," published in the Work in Progress series of the Stone Center at Wellesley College.

Cheryl Glickauf-Hughes, PhD, is an associate professor in the Department of Psychology at Georgia State University and an adjunct professor at Emory University School of Medicine; she also has a private practice in Atlanta, Georgia. Dr. Glickauf-Hughes has written numerous articles in the areas of object relations theory, personality disorders, and supervision, as well as a book with Marolyn Wells, *Treatment of the Masochistic Personality: An Interactional–Object Relations Approach to Psychotherapy* (Jason Aronson, 1995). She is currently completing a second book with Dr. Wells, *Object Relations Therapy: An Interactional Approach to Psychoanalytic Treatment* (Jason Aronson, in press).

Judith Horton, PhD, is the clinical director of the Mental Health/Mental Retardation Program at a state women's prison, and also maintains a private practice. She has been a clinician for 26 years, and received her doctorate in clinical psychology from Georgia State University in 1994. Her interests and expertise are in personality disorders, self-esteem, and women's issues.

Suzanne Imes, PhD, is a psychologist in independent practice in Atlanta, specializing in body-oriented Gestalt therapy with individuals, couples, and groups. She is an adjunct assistant professor of psychology at Georgia State University, where she supervises advanced clinical psychology graduate students. She is cofounder and director of the Gestalt Institute of Georgia, a fellow of the Georgia Psychological Association (GPA), and a former chair of the Women's Division of the GPA.

Les Kertay, PhD, received his doctorate in clinical psychology from Georgia State University in 1995 and has been a certified practitioner of Rolfing structural integration since 1979. He has a long-standing interest in the area of body–mind therapies and has been actively engaged in research in the field. He has recently begun several consultation groups intended to help health care professionals incorporate a knowledge of psychological dynamics and ethics into their practices. He is currently in private practice in Atlanta, Georgia.

Suzann Smith Lawry, PhD, is a graduate of the clinical psychology program at Georgia State University. She has specialized in women's issues and sexual abuse for the past 8 years; she has worked with both sexually abused children and adults as well as conducting research with victims and offenders. She has provided workshops at local, state, and national conferences and in-service training sessions on a variety of topics, including the use of creativity in healing from childhood sexual abuse. She is currently in private practice in Atlanta, Georgia.

David Mandelbaum, PhD, received his doctorate in human development and family studies from Pennsylvania State University in 1975. He taught for 6 years at Elmira College in Elmira, New York, and developed and implemented its first counseling center, directing it for 2 years. Currently he is in private practice in Wilmington, Delaware, and is known for his work with children and adolescents. In addition, he incorporates Gestalt therapy and Gestalt body work in his therapy with adolescents and adults. He has received extensive training in the existential–Gestalt approach and in Gestalt body work with Edward W. L. Smith.

Judy Milakovich, PhD, has been in private practice for 17 years. Currently, she is the codirector of the Center for Psychotherapy and Life Skills Development, a large group private practice. She specializes in working with adults who are resolving trauma-related issues. She has trained in body-centered therapy with Edward W. L. Smith, Jack Rosenberg, and Malcolm and Katherine Brown.

Vicki J. Petras, BS, is pursuing a PhD in clinical psychology at Emory University. She graduated from Georgia State University with honors. She was the recipient of the 1996 Outstanding Psychology Undergraduate Award and was listed in the 1996 *Who's Who among College Students in American Universities and Colleges.* In addition, she received the 1996 PSI CHI Regional Research Award for presenting her honors thesis, "The Intent–Lethality Relation in Urban Adolescent Suicide Attempts," at Southeastern Psychological Association (SEPA). She is also involved in numerous activities, such as writing for the *News for GSU Psychology Majors,* serving as treasurer for PSI CHI: The National Honor Society in Psychology and as director of communications for the Mortar Board National Honor Society; and conducting research for the Grady Adolescent Suicide Project.

Susan L. Reviere, PhD, is involved in various research projects concerning psychological trauma, and is also the author of a book, *Memory of Childhood Trauma: A Clinician's Guide to the Literature* (Guilford Press, 1996). She works with a community mental health center in Atlanta, Georgia.

Alma Smith Silverthorn, PhD, received her doctorate in psychology from Georgia State University in 1970. After serving as an assistant professor in the Department of Psychiatry, University of Tennessee Medical School, and becoming an avid pilot, her 21 years of practice in Palo Alto, California, focused upon people of diverse ethnic backgrounds. This crystallized her interest in cross-cultural psychotherapy. She has published in *Voices* and *The Psychotherapy Patient.*

Edward W. L. Smith, PhD, ABPP, is a professor of psychology and Coordinator of Clinical Training at Georgia Southern University. His books include *The Growing Edge of Gestalt Therapy* (Brunner/Mazel, 1976; Citadel, 1977), *The Body in Psychotherapy* (McFarland, 1985), *Sexual Aliveness* (McFarland, 1987), *Not Just Pumping Iron: On the Psychology of Lifting Weights* (Charles C Thomas, 1989), and *Gestalt Voices*

(Ablex, 1992). He has offered professional training in psychotherapy throughout the United States and in Canada, the Caribbean, Europe, and Mexico. He is a former chair of the Training Committee of the American Academy of Psychotherapists, and a fellow of the GPA and the American Psychological Association (Divisions 29, 32, and 42). He has received a diploma in clinical psychology from the ABPP.

Pamela Torraco, MSW, received her BA from Wittenberg University and her master's degree from the University of Michigan. With experience in public health, hospital psychiatry, and outpatient treatment of children, she now practices long-term intensive psychotherapy with Dr. Reuven Bar-Levav and Associates, PC, in Southfield, Michigan. She and several other colleagues assisted Dr. Bar-Levav in developing his unified theory of general human motivation and behavior, presented by Dr. Bar-Levav in *Thinking in the Shadow of Feelings: A New Understanding of the Hidden Forces That Shape Individuals and Societies* (Simon & Schuster, 1988). The psychotherapy model according to which they practice aims at ego boundary repair and the working through of preverbal fear and rage. Ms. Torraco has authored several articles in professional journals, and has presented lectures and workshops at local, national, and international conferences. She is the current president as well as a senior faculty member of the Bar-Levav Educational Association, which provides postgraduate training in intensive psychotherapy. Ms. Torraco is a past president of the Michigan Group Psychotherapy Society, and is currently a member of the editorial board of the *International Journal of Psychotherapy and Critical Thought*.

PREFACE

Shrouded for many in a cloak of fear, rumor, and misinformation, touch is perhaps the most controversial topic in psychotherapy today. The professional literature is replete both with warnings of the risks therapists take when they touch clients, and with claims that any benefits of touch are only hypothetical or anecdotal. In response to this, many therapists express fear of being misunderstood if they touch clients and then of being vulnerable to ethical or even legal charges.

Such fear is spawned in large part, we believe, by lack of accurate information. There are many examples of simplification and distortion in the discussions of touch in psychotherapy. "Rules" designed for all therapists with all clients in all contexts are the ultimate of such simplification and distortion. We must not fall prey to such assumption of uniformity across therapists (of different personalities, theoretical orientations, and levels of experience), across clients (of different personalities, pathological mechanisms, and levels of consciousness), or across contexts (of different occasions, circumstances, and stages of therapy).

In the present volume, we have sought to begin to lift the cloak of misinformation about touch in psychotherapy. To do so, we have enlisted experts in the area of touch in psychotherapy to write of what they know. These theoreticians, researchers, and practitioners share in the pages that follow formulations and informed opinions gleaned from years of clinical experience. These, in turn, have been submitted to reflective critical thinking. Some of the authors also share empirical data generated from their research.

As editors, we have invited contributors based on their interest in the subject, their clinical or research expertise, and their varied approaches to the use of touch in psychotherapy. Although we have not attempted to be exhaustive in our representation of all possible personal or theoretical viewpoints, we have included several theoretical perspectives in order to provide a multifaceted view of how, when, and with whom touch may be used in the healing process. We chose not to represent the position that touch should never be used.

This book is divided into three sections, each of which reflect an aspect of the book's subtitle. The first section, "Theoretical and Ethical Considerations," provides a history, context, and rationale for the use of touch in psychotherapy, and lays the foundation for the ethical use of touch. The case is made that balanced and judicious use of touch should be acceptable in practice and open for scientific study.

In Chapter 1, "Traditions of Touch in Psychotherapy," Edward W. L. Smith offers a brief history of the use of touch from the early years of psychoanalysis to the present. Within the historical perspective, he suggests two sources for some of the bias encountered against touch in psychotherapy.

In Chapter 2, "Touch in Context," Les Kertay and Susan L. Reviere discuss touch as a fundamental form of communication. They point out that the decision to apply or withhold touch should be determined by the meaning of the touch, which in turn is examined in light of three contexts in which the touch occurs.

In Chapter 3, "A Taxonomy and Ethics of Touch in Psychotherapy," Smith presents one possible classification system for types of touch. He develops a decision-making model that involves using both ethical and theoretical guidelines.

Chapter 4, which completes the first section, is Reuven Bar-Levav's "A Rationale for Physical Touching in Psychotherapy." He makes a compelling case for the corrective impact of touch on "the scared infant within the adult patient."

The second section, "Research Perspectives," includes research on the communicability of touch, touch from the therapist's perspective, and touch from the client's perspective.

In Chapter 5, Joen Fagan and Alma Smith Silverthorn write about "Research on Communication by Touch." They demonstrate that people are able to discriminate among many different types of touch. This ability to understand emotional communication from others through touch is an important component of emotional well-being.

Next, Judy Milakovich identifies factors that differentiate therapists who do touch from those who do not touch their clients in individual psychotherapy. She describes her research results in Chapter 6, "Differences between Therapists Who Touch and Those Who Do Not."

Pauline Rose Clance and Vicki J. Petras report both quantitative and qualitative findings in Chapter 7, "Therapists' Recall of Their Decision-Making Processes Regarding the Use of Touch in Ongoing Psychotherapy: A Preliminary Study."

In Chapter 8, "The Experience of Nonerotic Physical Contact in Traditional Psychotherapy," Pamela Geib presents qualitative data from the clients' perspective. From her research, she has derived five factors that affect people's experience of touch in psychotherapy; she discusses four of them here.

Using the four of Geib's factors discussed in Chapter 8, Judith Horton and her colleagues have investigated touch from the clients' perspective. Horton reports the results of this survey in Chapter 9, "Further Research on the Patient's Experience of Touch in Therapy."

The third section, "Insights from Practice," allows the reader to enter the experience of touch in therapy from the perspective of therapists and/or clients. The material in this section is generally either care-centered or autobiographical.

In Chapter 10, "Thoughts on Using Touch in Psychotherapy," Joen Fagan uses a case study to explicate principles and guidelines for the use of touch in psychotherapy. These are derived from the wisdom of long clinical experience.

Cheryl Glickauf-Hughes and Susan Chance distinguish clients for whom the use of touch in psychotherapy can be useful from those for whom touch may be harmful. This material constitutes Chapter 11, "An Individualized and Interactive Object Relations Perspective on the Use of Touch in Psychotherapy."

By contrast, a Gestalt therapy perspective is articulated in Chapter 12, "Long-Term Clients' Experience of Touch in Gestalt Therapy." Suzanne Imes weaves her therapeutic perspective into case studies of clients who have been extensively, moderately, and minimally touched.

In Chapter 13, Suzann Smith Lawry addresses the issue of touch with sexually abused clients. In "Touch and Clients Who Have Been Sexually Abused," the author demonstrates the therapeutic usefulness of touch with such clients, without losing sight of precautionary measures a clinician needs to consider.

In an autobiographical mode, David Mandelbaum, in Chapter 14, shares "The Impact of Physical Touch on Professional Development." He describes his experiences in several professional training contexts.

In the final chapter, Pamela Torraco makes the reader privy to the inner process of a therapist's using touch with several clients over a long period of time in her career. This chapter is titled "Jean's Legacy: On the Use of Physical Touch in Long-Term Psychotherapy." From her extensive clinical experience, she distills 11 guidelines for the use of touch in therapy.

One who reads all the chapters of this book will encounter overlap in opinion, as well as disagreement on when, where, how, and under what circumstances clients most benefit from touch in therapy. All agree that touch should never be sexual in nature, and that touch needs to be used with care, respect, and caution within the context of overall good psychotherapy. We applaud these therapists, as well as others not represented here, who are giving professional energy and attention to this important subject.

We also commend Barbara Watkins, Senior Editor at The Guilford Press, for her encouragement throughout our pursuit of this book. Her thoughtful input and meticulous editing have greatly enhanced the quality of *Touch in Psychotherapy: Theory, Research, and Practice.*

EDWARD W. L. SMITH
PAULINE ROSE CLANCE
SUZANNE IMES

CONTENTS

TOUCH IN PSYCHOTHERAPY

I

THEORETICAL AND ETHICAL CONSIDERATIONS

1

TRADITIONS OF TOUCH IN PSYCHOTHERAPY

Edward W. L. Smith

The use of touch in healing has ancient roots in magico-religious and shamanic practices. Given these roots, it is no surprise that the "laying on of hands" and other forms of touch were handed down to modern healers. Various forms of touch have been in the repertoire of health-care workers since their emergence from the realms of religion and magic. Whether for diagnosis or treatment, physicians, nurses, athletic trainers, and of course massage therapists have put touch to use. As a healing art, psychotherapy too inherited the tradition of touch. Prior to the emergence of psychoanalysis, psychiatric treatments consisted mostly of physical interventions, including the use of touch (Levitan & Johnson, 1986; Wilson, 1982).

Surprisingly, this tradition of touch is apparently either misunderstood or totally unknown by many contemporary psychotherapists. Take, for example, the statement by Kilburg (1988) in the leading psychotherapy journal of the American Psychological Association. In reference to what he terms "physical interventions," most of which involve "some degree of touching," he states, "The techniques are relatively new to the practice of psychology" (p. 516). Yet the history of psychotherapy informs us clearly that touch has been a part of the activity from its emergence as an identifiable entity.

Although a traditional part of psychotherapy, touch continues to

3

be a focus of controversy. Why is this so? Concerns about touch in psychotherapy have been raised by many. These concerns may be theoretical, as in the traditional psychoanalytic position, may be ethical, or may be political. The ethical concern seems to reduce to a fear that touch will lead to inappropriate, therapist-need-serving, exploitative touch, such as sexual touch. In the realm of gender politics, Alyn (1988) has from a feminist position raised concern about the use of touch by a male therapist as having a disempowering effect on a female patient, given that touching in a social setting often defines power. All of these concerns demand to be taken seriously. Based on appropriate consideration of these concerns, as well as further theoretical considerations such as when touch is contraindicated even within one of the camps which support and legitimize touch in psychotherapy, one may choose not to touch. Likewise, personal discomfort with touch on the part of the therapist would, in general, contraindicate touching a patient.

I believe, however, that more complex reasons also keep the topic of touch in the realm of controversy. I suggest that the controversy is kept alive through bias against touch born of an implicit Western cultural philosophy and born of historical influences and context. I explore each of these sources of this controversy-producing bias or prejudice in turn.

SOURCES OF THE BIAS AGAINST TOUCH IN PSYCHOTHERAPY

Mind–Body Dualism

First, I suggest that the prejudice against touching in psychotherapy is a by-product of the mind–body dichotomy so well entrenched in the philosophical underpinning of Western society. This dualistic thinking is deeply rooted in our culture. As clearly stated by Descartes, Western culture has tended to separate, conceptually, *res cogitans* (things mental) from *res extensa* (things physical). From this philosophical heritage have come the dualistic sciences that we have today. In the realm of psychological problems, many couch the question of etiology in these terms: "Is it physical or mental?" Even professionals follow the same dualistic bias in asking, "Is it organic or functional?" Such "either–or" thinking leads to a diagnosis that places a disorder in the hands of either a "*physic*-ian" or a "*psycho*-therapist." This paradigm has clear implications for treatment. If the problem is a physical one (i.e., organic, genetic), then the soma needs to be treated, logically, by *physical* means. But if the problem is a "mental" one, then the psyche requires that *mental* means be used. What I am proposing is that this nonholistic paradigm makes it difficult to think in terms of physical intervention as part of psychotherapy. If, on the other hand, one subscribes to a more organismic or holistic view, then therapeutic interventions can be judged on their own merit, free from dualistic bias. It is this dualistic bias, I suggest, that hampers open and clear thinking about the legitimate place of touch in psychotherapy.

Historical Influences and Context

Second, I believe that the prejudice against touching in psychotherapy is the heritage of historical influences that came in time to be taken as scientifically based truth. I allude to a number of contingencies in the life and work of Sigmund Freud.

Freud (1923/1960) stated that the ego is "first and foremost body-ego." In this, he was acknowledging that experience of ego develops as experience of body. Or, as he wrote (Freud, 1923/1960), "the ego is ultimately derived from bodily sensations, chiefly from those springing from the surface of the body. It may thus be regarded as a mental projection of the surface of the body" (p. 16).

The important developmental implication of this view is that the lack of certain body sensations will limit ego development. That is to say, to the extent that a child does not have certain body experiences, the child will not develop ego in that realm and will have an ego deficit. For example, if the parenting figures do not provide adequate experience for the child in being held securely, supported against gravity, then the child will have a deficiency in the self-support function. Picking up, laying down, holding, and rocking the child, all with firm and steady support, will provide the body with sensations of support that can be incorporated in the growth of the child's ego. The person who is bereft of such body experience as a child may thus be deficient in adult life in the egoic experience of self-support (Smith, 1985). Moreover, the usual "talking therapies" may be insufficient to redress such a deficiency:

> There is a profound therapeutic implication to all of this—if the person has an ego deficiency because of inadequate ego-forming body experiences, then analysis and insight into the problem will be inadequate to bring about change. For change to come about means to provide body experiences which are ego-developing. Psychotherapy, in such situations, would need to provide the opportunity for the patient to have an adequate amount of the experiences which were inadequately present in the previous learning history. Put simply, ego growth and development come about through experiential learning, not from analyzing. (Smith, 1985, pp. 3–4)

What I see in Freud's statements is his laying the groundwork for a psychotherapy that would rely heavily on touch in order to provide ego-building experiences. The developmental and therapeutic implications of Freud's view of the ego as a "body-ego" provide a theoretical rationale for using touch in psychotherapy.

Later clinical and laboratory research provided evidence and conclusions that are consistent with Freud's view of ego development. Harlow (1958; Harlow, Harlow, & Levin, 1957), for instance, in his now-classic studies with rhesus monkeys, provided evidence that physical contact between mother and infant is crucial for the healthy development of the latter. Also classic is the work of Spitz (1957) with human infants and mothers, showing modes of physical interaction that lead to mental health or to disturbance in the development and differentiation of a sense of self. The role of parental touch in the development of body image and love for self and others has been described at length by such writers as Erikson (1950), Hoffer (1950), and Anna Freud (1965). Mahler and McDevitt (1982) have stated with considerable poignancy that touch experience "seems to be the condition on which the feeling of being alive rests" (p. 833). The importance of touch and the deleterious effects of lack of touch as suggested by research have been documented in a thoroughgoing volume by Montagu (1971), which he entitled *Touching*.

The list of clinicians and researchers who have emphasized the importance of touch in the normal development of the self or ego is extensive; I have alluded to this literature only briefly, in order to make the point that Freud can now be seen as on solid ground in his view of the developmental importance of touch. There are several worthy reviews of the relevant literature to which an interested reader can turn. Among these are the reviews found in "To Touch or Not to Touch" (Goodman & Teicher, 1988), "The Vitalizing and the Revitalizing Experience of Reliability: The Place of Touch in Psychotherapy" (Kupfermann & Smaldino, 1987), "Regressive Work as a Therapeutic Treatment" (Smith, 1990), "Are Psychotherapists Out of Touch?" (Woodmansey, 1988), and more recently "The Use of Touch in Psychotherapy: Theoretical and Ethical Considerations" (Kertay & Reviere, 1993; parts of Chapter 2 of this volume are loosely based on this article). In addition, several other chapters in the present volume review selected portions of the literature on touch in psychotherapy.

Returning to Freud's work, one can find a further rationale for the use of touch in psychotherapy. In a letter to Wilhelm Fliess in 1899, Freud wrote, "From time to time I visualize a second part of the method of treatment—provoking patients' feelings as well as their ideas, as if that were quite indispensable" (quoted in Lowen, 1971, p. xi). This "second part of treatment," the provocation of affect, implies the use of touch; although talking can, of course, provoke feeling, the most direct access to affect involves manipulation of the body (Smith, 1985). "In fact, in the early development of psychoanalysis, touch was occasionally used to help patients express their feelings. Freud, for example, in his early work with hysteria, used massage to the neck and head to facilitate emotional expression and age regression in his patients, while also allowing them to touch him (Forer, 1969; Levitan & Johnson, 1986; Wilson, 1982)" (Kertay & Reviere, 1993, p. 33).

Given Freud's insight concerning the importance of touch in ego development and his laying the groundwork for the use of touch in psychotherapy, and given that touch was an established part of psychiatric treatment prior to the advent of psychoanalysis, what happened to create the controversy around touch? Perhaps Freud wanted not to be associated with the methods used in psychiatry before his "talking cure." We know that he was very keen on scientific respectability for psychoanalysis; this may have been one reason not to touch, out of concern for being associated with prescientific "laying on of hands." Given his historical context (Victorian Vienna), Freud lived and worked in a society beset with sexual prudery. Surely such prudery also gave Freud caution as he developed his theories of psychosexual stages of development, childhood sexuality, and the sexual etiology of neurosis. Surely, too, the case of Anna O., in which Breuer and Freud encountered the incorporation of Breuer in Anna's recovery of incestuous memories, gave both men serious pause. Perhaps this was a specific reason to abandon touch.

Freud did not focus on the early phases of infant development, but placed his emphasis on the Oedipal period. His emphasis was on the drives (at different periods in his theorizing, sex or Eros, aggression, and death or Thanatos) rather than on developmental needs. It followed from this focus that he cautioned the analyst not to gratify the patient's needs, lest such gratification take the patient's energy away from the primary task of analysis. Gratifying the patient's needs, as touching would presumably do, was also thought to interfere with transference. The task in classical psychoanalysis, developed about 1913–1914, is to make unconscious material conscious by means of free association and the analysis of the transference. In order to be able to accomplish the final goal—that is, resolution of the transference neurosis—the therapist needs to take the role of the "blank screen" throughout the analytic treatment. That is, the analyst needs to be impersonal and nonevaluative, avoiding any action that could contaminate the transference.

Freud's concerns about touch may well have been overdetermined, involving all of the considerations mentioned above. But perhaps his greatest personal concern was not theoretical. In his confrontation of Sandor Ferenczi for the latter's use of nurturant touch in order to help patients tolerate the pain which was avoided by means of characterological defenses, Freud expressed deep concern for the image of psychoanalysis as well as its dogma. Freud wrote a letter to Ferenczi asking where the latter would stop:

> A number of independent thinkers in the matter of technique will say to themselves: why stop? Certainly one gets further when one adopts "pawing" as well. . . . And then bolder ones will come along who will go further to peeping and showing, and soon we shall have accepted in the techniques of analysis the whole repertoire of . . . petting parties, resulting in an enormous increase of interest in psychoanalysis among both analysts and patients. (quoted in Jones, 1955, p. 163)

Clearly, orthodox psychoanalysis no longer had room for analysts who touched. Contingencies in Freud's life led to a dogma, a doctrine forbidding touch. In time, this dogma led some to a taboo against touch in psychotherapy.

Most conservative psychoanalytic systems look upon touch as outside the purview of psychoanalytic treatment. In these views, not only is it not of use, but it is contraindicated; any touch may interfere with the transference, as well as provide fulfillment of infantile desires in need of being analyzed. One does not need to search far in the literature even now to find authoritative voices that are adamant in this regard.

CONTINUING TRADITIONS OF TOUCH IN THERAPY SETTINGS

In spite of the strong bias (and even prejudice, in some quarters) against touch in psychotherapy, it is and always has been present in the therapy setting. Notwithstanding the dualistic thinking born of the mind–body dichotomy in Western philosophy, as well as the bias of classical drive-focused (or id-focused) psychoanalysis, there is a continuing tradition of touch in psychotherapy. There are those who support the ethical and judicious use of certain forms of touch as legitimate and, under some circumstances, indispensable. Such support is found in three distinct camps: in certain psychodynamic theories; in Reichian and neo-Reichian theories; and in humanistic psychology. I discuss each of these briefly in turn, and also add a short postscript on approaches involving role play.

Psychodynamic Traditions of Touch

As discussed earlier, Freud laid the groundwork for touch in psycho-therapy in his view that the ego is first and foremost a "body-ego." But Freud's emphasis was on the drives, the id. Later analysts began focusing on the ego and its development. In so doing, they found the traditional techniques of analysis inadequate for treating certain types of patients. With patients who had pre-Oedipal problems, techniques through which the patients were allowed to regress were found to be more effective. This approach gave rise, then, to holding, rocking, or even bottle feeding. Thus, various modes of touch were admitted into psychodynamic work, with various analysts differing on their level of caution. For instance, Sponitz (1972) recommended touching only in situations where it actually furthers the analysis of transference. Taking a less cautious stance, Mintz (1969) endorsed touch as an expression of nurturance or support, while still opposing its use for the gratifica-tion of infantile needs when this would interfere with growth. But she stated (Mintz, 1973) that "when contact seems natural . . . the question may be asked as to whether the transference may not be more contaminated by its avoidance than by its presence" (p. 185). "Probably there are times when a psychotic patient needs physical holding," Winnicott (1965, p. 240) concluded.

The recognition of the important difference between "drive" needs and developmental needs led to modifications in the traditional psycho-analytic technique. And the modifications included the use of touch. Among the ego analysts and the object relations analysts, we find many examples of the judicious use of touch based on clinical experience as well as carefully thought-out theoretical rationales (and, of course, ethical considerations). The expansion of the use of touch in the psychodynamic therapies included its use with various populations—patients with Oedi-pal character structures (neurotic), as well as those with pre-Oedipal character structures (psychotic and character-disordered).

Reichian and Neo-Reichian Traditions of Touch

The second camp in which the use of touch in psychotherapy is given support is that of the Reichian and neo-Reichian therapists. These posi-tions are rooted again in the work of Freud, as noted earlier. To reiterate, Freud wrote, "From time to time I visualize a second part of the method of treatment—provoking patients' feelings as well as their ideas, as if that were quite indispensable" (quoted in Lowen, 1971, p. xi). It was Ferenczi who followed Freud's lead. In response to the lack of therapeutic impact of the traditional psychoanalytic technique on certain psychological problems that seemed to have their genesis in pre-Oedipal events, Ferenczi developed what he termed "activity techniques." He experimented with relaxation exercises, patient self-restraints from fidgeting, and so forth, as well as with touch. The importance of his activity techniques was summarized by Ferenczi in 1919:

> The fact that the expression of emotion or motor actions forced from the patients evoke secondarily memories from the unconscious rests partly on the reciprocity of affect and idea emphasized by Freud. . . . The awakening of a memory can—as in catharsis—bring an emotional reaction with it, but an activity enacted from the patient, or an emotion set at freedom, can equally well expose the repressed ideas associated with such processes. (quoted in Lowen, 1971, pp. 10–11)

Ferenczi's work was being guided by the new therapeutic paradigm which he was pioneering. In the old paradigm, talking leads to memories of important childhood events, and those memories lead to feelings (affect, catharsis); in the new one, manipulation of the body leads directly to feelings and the childhood memories following the affect. It was Ferenczi's student Wilhelm Reich who developed the techniques that demonstrated the great therapeutic power of this new paradigm. Concerning the paradigm, Reich (1942/1973) wrote that body interventions offer "the possibility of avoiding, when necessary, the complicated detour via the psychic structure and of breaking through to the affects directly from the somatic attitude. In this way, the repressed affect appears before the corresponding remembrance" (p. 301).

Reich adopted and developed a model of therapy involving strong catharsis. He stated that "the effects of a psychic experience are determined not by its content, but by the amount of vegetative energy which is mobilized by the experience" (Reich, 1942/1973, p. 316). Maintaining that affect and expression can be held at bay by means of chronic muscular tensions, Reich introduced the concept of defenses as total organismic functions:

> Central to Reich's (1949) position, and perhaps his most important theoretical contribution, was the concept of the "muscular armor." Reich suggested that the neurotic solution of the infantile instinctual conflict (the chronic conflict between instinctual demands on the one hand and the counterdemands of the social world) is brought about through a generalized alteration of functioning which ultimately crystallizes into a neurotic "character" . . . This "character" is, then, essentially a narcissistic protective mechanism, originally formed for protection against punishment of the child's instinctual expression by the parents or other agents of the social order. It is retained for

protection against instinctual "dangers" from within. Character is an organismic phenomenon, manifesting on the physical plane as chronic muscular rigidities. These chronic muscular rigidities, or muscular armor, serve to negate or block impulses to action which are inconsistent with the neurotic character. In time, the muscular armor serves to bind free-floating anxiety. (Smith, 1985, pp. 5–6)

Consistent with his theoretical position, and on the basis of clinical observations, Reich developed both diagnostic methods and therapeutic interventions involving touch. In his view, given that the character of the patient is manifested in the muscular armor, the therapist can diagnose the patient by means of palpating the muscles to discern the pattern of muscular tensions. Thus, Reich touched to diagnose. Given Reich's position (earlier stated by Freud) that remembrances, in order to be curative, must be accompanied by appropriate affect, and that muscular armor can hold at bay both affect and expression, Reich developed methods for softening the muscular armor. One such method, "orgonomic massage," involves strategic application of brief, heavy pressure to armored muscles. When the method is used successfully, the affect that had been blocked is released—often dramatically, and often with concomitant lifting of repression, or at least clearer and more vivified memories. (Such "body work" is described in detail in my book *The Body in Psychotherapy* [Smith, 1985].) The important point here is that Reich introduced, or at least systematized, forms of touch for psychodiagnosis and psychotherapy. With Reich, certain forms of touch became the techniques themselves.

Reich was therapist, supervisor, or trainer to several people who developed therapy positions in their own right. A "neo-Reichian" tradition ensued. Fritz Perls, the major founder of Gestalt therapy, was an analysand and later trainee of Reich. Although he did not incorporate Reich's formalized touch techniques such as orgonomic massage into Gestalt therapy, his work includes many examples of touching and being touched by patients. Some who trained with Reich later than Perls did either incorporated Reich's formal techniques or developed techniques of their own involving the formal use of touch. Examples abound. Elsworth Baker continued Reich's work in the United States, while Ola Raknes did so in Norway. David Boadella made some modifications in Reich's work in England. In the United States, Alexander Lowen and John Pierrakos developed bioenergetics; Charles Kelley developed Radix (and coined the term "neo-Reichian"). More recently, Pierrakos revised his work under the name of core energetics. Influenced both by Lowen and by Raknes, Malcolm Brown developed the positions of direct body contact psychotherapy and (later, with his wife, Katherine Ennis Brown) organismic psychotherapy. (These are only the most notable of the traditions. For an overview of each of these positions, and a comparison of them, I refer the reader again to *The Body in Psychotherapy* [Smith, 1985].)

The Reichian tradition has many branches and represents a large number of practitioners throughout the world. The major point for present purposes is that in this tradition touch is not only legitimized; it is a major mode through which the therapist interacts with the patient. In this tradition, touch is formalized and elevated into systematized techniques.

Humanistic Traditions of Touch

The third camp in which touch in psychotherapy is supported is that of humanistic psychotherapies. Compared to the positions of the psychodynamic and Reichian traditions, the humanistic position on touch is less theoretically complex. Touch is not formalized, as in the Reichian tradition; nor is it of concern because it might interface with transference and motivation, as in the psychodynamic positions. Rather, it is viewed as a natural and spontaneous expression of genuine (nontransferential) relationship. Open, honest expression, highly valued in humanistic psychotherapy, can be served through this natural medium of communication.

Born of the humanistic movement (or, as it soon became known, the human potential movement), encounter groups encouraged experimentation with touch, among other ways of relating and communicating. The emphasis was on openness, honesty, spontaneity, and genuineness. There was a trust that whatever came up could be processed, as long as these values prevailed. The encounter group finally blended into psychotherapy in general, influencing many therapists and having an impact on therapy as a whole. Influenced by humanistic psychology—with its reaction against what it perceived as the bias toward pathology in psychoanalysis, and the partitive concepts and dehumanizing effects of behavior therapy—many therapists pushed (and continue to push) for genuine person-to-person encounters. In such contexts, touch certainly has a place.

In practice, the lines between the three camps described above are often more conceptual than real. Many therapists consider themselves eclectic; as such, they integrate theory, techniques, or both from these three camps that provide a place for touch in psychotherapy, as well as from a more traditional psychoanalytic stance that would prohibit touch.

Postscript: Approaches Involving Role Play

Also important to recognize are therapy approaches that involve role play, and therefore often involve touching. When role play is done in a group setting, such as in psychodrama or Pesso–Boyden system psychomotor (PBSP) therapy, the therapist is in the role of directing the drama, and touch involves the group members who are enacting specifically defined roles. The actual words used and actions taken by the "actors" may be more or less closely directed by the therapist/director. In psychodrama the actors may be given more license to improvise, whereas in PBSP therapy, the actors tend to be much more highly scripted by the therapist/director in close consultation with the patients. In either case, the therapist is directing and therefore either encouraging or discouraging touch among the participants in the drama—patients and those who agree to take part in the drama for the benefit of the "patient." At times PBSP sessions are held one on one with a therapist. At such times, the therapist may enroll himself or herself as a figure in the drama, and thus may be in physical contact with the patient. So, with role-play therapies, touch is again legitimized as a procedure to be considered. (For an overview of the theory and procedures of PBSP therapy, see the discussion of psychomotor therapy in *The Body in Psychotherapy* [Smith, 1985].)

CONCLUSION

The major thesis of this chapter is that touch has been part of psychotherapy from its inchoate beginnings until the present. Touch in psychotherapy can be found as a strategic means of encouraging regression and providing nurturance or support; as a formalized and systematized body of technical interventions in the service of characterological growth through elicitation and expression of affect; or as a genuine human expression of person-to-person relating. Many therapies include it as legitimate praxis when used ethically and appropriately, as defined by their theory.

Several surveys of practitioners have indicated that touch in psychotherapy is quite common. In a recent survey of members of the American Academy of Psychotherapists, Tirnauer, Smith, and Foster (1996) reported that only 13% of those in the survey indicated that they "never touch" patients.

It is apparent that touch has always been a part of psychotherapy, and it seems likely that it will continue to be so. The remainder of this book is devoted to exploring the factors involved in its appropriate use.

REFERENCES

Alyn, J. (1988). The politics of touch in therapy: A reply to Willison and Masson. *Journal of Counseling and Development, 66,* 432–433.

Erikson, E. (1950). *Childhood and society.* New York: Norton.

Forer, B. R. (1969). The taboo against touching in psychotherapy. *Psychotherapy: Theory, Research, and Practice, 6*(4), 229–231.

Freud, A. (1965). *Normality and pathology in childhood.* New York: International Universities Press.

Freud, S. (1960). *The ego and the id* (J. Strachey, Ed. and Trans.). New York: Norton. (Original work published 1923)

Goodman, M., & Teicher, A. (1988). To touch or not to touch. *Psychotherapy, 25*(4), 492–500.

Harlow, H. (1958). The nature of love. *American Psychologist, 13,* 673–685.

Harlow, H., Harlow, M., & Levin, H. (1957). *Patterns of child rearing.* White Plains, NY: Row, Peterson.

Hoffer, W. (1950). The development of the body ego. *Psychoanalytic Study of the Child, 5,* 18–23.

Jones, E. (1955). *The life and work of Sigmund Freud: Vol. 2. Years of maturity.* New York: Basic Books.

Kertay, L., & Reviere, S. L. (1993). The use of touch in psychotherapy: Theoretical and ethical considerations. *Psychotherapy, 30*(1), 32–40.

Kilburg, R. (1988). Psychologists and physical interventions: Ethics, standards, and legal implications. *Psychotherapy, 25*(4), 516–531.

Kupfermann, K., & Smaldino, C. (1987). The vitalizing and the revitalizing experience of reliability: The place of touch in psychotherapy. *Clinical Social Work Journal, 15*(3), 223–235.

Levitan, A., & Johnson, J. (1986). The role of touch in healing and hypnotherapy. *American Journal of Clinical Hypnosis, 28*(4), 218–223.

Lowen, A. (1971). *The language of the body.* New York: Collier.

Mahler, M., & McDevitt, J. (1982). Thoughts on the emergence of the sense of self, with particular emphasis on the body self. *Journal of the American Psychoanalytic Association, 30,* 827–848.

Mintz, E. (1969). On the rationale of touch in psychotherapy. *Psychotherapy, 6*(4), 232–234.

Mintz, E. (1973). On the rationale of touch in psychotherapy. In E. Hendrick & M. Ruitenbeck (Eds.), *The analytic situation: How patient and therapist communicate.* Chicago: Aldine.

Montagu, A. (1971). *Touching: The human significance of the skin.* New York: Columbia University Press.

Reich, W. (1949). *Character analysis.* New York: Noonday Press.

Reich, W. (1973). *The function of the orgasm.* New York: Simon & Schuster. (Original work published 1942)

Smith, E. (1985). *The body in psychotherapy.* Jefferson, NC: McFarland.

Smith, S. (1990). Regressive work as a therapeutic treatment. *Transactional Analysis Journal, 20*(4), 253–262.

Spitz, R. (1957). *No and yes.* New York: International Universities Press.

Sponitz, H. (1972). Touch countertransference in group psychotherapy. *International Journal of Group Psychotherapy, 22,* 455–463.

Tirnauer, L., Smith, E., & Foster, P. (1996). The American Academy of Psychotherapists Research Committee Survey of members. *Voices, 32*(2), 87–94.

Wilson, J. (1982). The value of touch in psychotherapy. *American Journal of Orthopsychiatry, 52*(1), 65–72.

Winnicott, D. (1965). *The maturational processes and the facilitating environment.* New York: International Universities Press.

Woodmansey, A. (1988). Are psychotherapists out of touch? *British Journal of Psychotherapy, 5*(1), 57–65.

2

TOUCH IN CONTEXT

Les Kertay
Susan L. Reviere

Touch is a fundamental, multilayered, and powerful form of communication thought to be essential to normative human development. No more and no less than other modalities of conveying both feeling and meaning, it can contribute to growth, and it can contribute to healing where growth has been disrupted. However, touch can also, when misused, create harm. Thus, in many different realms—professional ethics panels, state licensing boards, malpractice insurers, and the courts—practitioners in the healing professions, particularly psychotherapists, are increasingly faced with compelling questions concerning ethical, legal, and theoretical responsibilities in the therapeutic use of touch. Given the increased interest in touch-oriented therapies in Western culture, what drives a renewed taboo against touch in psychotherapy? Is such a taboo indicated? Or are there circumstances in which touch can be appropriately employed in psychotherapy for the benefit of patients and without risk of injury?

In a previous review of the ethical and theoretical considerations surrounding the use of touch in psychotherapy, we argued that it is impossible simply to ignore these issues. We stated that "the question may not be whether or not therapists *should* touch their patients, but rather *how* touch is utilized and processed in therapy" (Kertay & Reviere, 1993, p. 39; italics in original). That is to say, if a therapist decides to touch a given patient, he or she must do so in a thoughtful manner and must be willing to accept responsibility for the patient's interpretation of the touch. Likewise, if the therapist decides not to touch, there must be a similar willingness to accept responsibility for the meanings that the patient will assign to the absence of a natural form of human contact.

Potential misuses and miscommunications notwithstanding, we believe that touch can be wisely and judiciously applied in the course of therapy, to the benefit of patients. We believe that the decision to apply or withhold touch in psychotherapy should be determined by the meaning of the touch, and that an interpretation of this meaning is determined in large part by the contexts in which touch occurs. In this chapter, we review some of the contextual cues to the meaning of touch. We refer to empirical findings in the literature related to various aspects of touch in psychotherapy, whenever such findings are available. When they are not, we comment on the nature of the contexts and their implications for using or withholding touch in a psychotherapy relationship.

DEVELOPMENTAL IMPLICATIONS OF TOUCH

Certain theoretical positions consider psychotherapy as a forum for continued development of self. Thus, as we consider the utility of touch in psychotherapy, it may first be helpful to consider its role in human development.

Touch is a critical and pervasive form of communication. Physical contact provides crucial physiological information about the environment throughout an organism's lifespan, and the skin functions in the regulation of internal homeostasis. In humans, the skin has acquired significance beyond physiology and has taken on social and psychological functions as well (Masters, 1987; Montagu, 1971). With these added functions, touch between human individuals becomes a means for communicating a vast range of meanings, which are influenced by the context in which the touch occurs.

Harlow (1958) demonstrated the importance of touch in the development of the young monkey, noting that the infant monkeys he studied required touch as much as food for their normal development. In fact, at times the monkeys preferred the comfort of tactile stimulation to food, even when they were hungry. Spitz (1945) extended these findings to humans in studies of the effects of touch deprivation on infants and children in orphanages. He demonstrated that infants deprived of physical contact failed to develop normally and became physically ill, despite adequate attention to their other physical needs.

Touch has additional importance in human development. Touch is the earliest form of communication between parent and child. Through touch, the parent provides orientation, comfort, and critical affective information to the child (Kupfermann & Smaldino, 1987; Levitan & Johnson, 1986; Wilson, 1982). The early psychological sense of self, and early self–other distinctions, are derived in part from early experiences of the presence or absence of touch and from the quality of that touch (Kupfermann & Smaldino, 1987; Mahler & McDevitt, 1982; Mahler, Pine, & Bergman, 1975). In fact, Kreuger (1989, 1990) has argued that the development of the psychological self depends primarily on parent–child interactions and attachments, which are governed by the physical contact that accompanies other forms of communication.

Numerous authors have tied the development of psychopathology of the self, particularly the schizoid, borderline, and narcissistic personality disorders, to deviant interactions between the child and his or her main nurturing figure (Horner, 1984, 1990; Kernberg, 1975, 1976; Kohut, 1971; Mahler, 1968; Winnicott, 1965). If we consider that touch is a primary mode of communication, bonding, and comfort between the primary caregiver and the infant or young child, we may infer that disordered or inappropriate experiences of touch constitute one source of subsequent disruptions in development. The relationship between developing personality disorders and problems with touch remains a theoretical construct with little empirical support (due in large part to the attendant problems in research methodology). However, other connections have been documented.

For example, the relationship between disordered touch sensation and a wide range of subsequent psychological problems was presented in a case study of a young male with congenitally absent somatic sensation (Dubovsky & Groban, 1975). In addition, a prospective study comparing preterm extremely low-birthweight (ELBW) infants with matched full-term controls was presented by Grunau, Whitfield, Petrie, and Fryer (1994). They found a higher incidence of pathological somatization in the ELBW infants who had been hospitalized the longest, and who were therefore subjected at an early age to repeated medical interventions as well as prolonged touch deprivation. Interestingly, these authors found that one of the factors that predicted high somatization scores at age $4\frac{1}{2}$ was a child's tendency to avoid touch or holding at age 3. Sivik (1993) also found a link among hypersensitivity to touch, somatization, and alexithymia.

Without appropriate experience of the sense of touch, it is difficult to develop a sense of one's body, and some authors argue that a sense of a "body self" is the ground of the psychological self. Schilder (1935),

Fisher (1970, 1986, 1990; Fisher & Cleveland, 1968), Shontz (1974, 1975, 1990), and others have placed a central emphasis on the sense of the physical self in the development and expression of the psychological self. Specific empirical support for the relationship between the body image and the experience of touch is available from a number of sources. For example, Gupta and Schork (1995) found an inverse relationship between perceived tactile nurturing during childhood and body dissatisfaction scores, as well as a positive correlation between current desire to receive nurturance and scores on a Drive for Thinness scale. They noted that their findings support the importance of nurturance—specifically, tactile nurturance—in the development of body image, especially among women. Finally, studies of motor development have demonstrated that milestones in the development of physical sensations appear to set timetables for the development of psychological functions (e.g., Bushnell & Boudreau, 1993), and, by extension, for the development of the psychological self as a whole. Thus, although recent empirical literature related to the issue of touch and development is rather sparse, the literature that exists demonstrates important connections that may have implications for understanding the role of touch in later development and healing.

EARLY TABOOS AGAINST TOUCH IN PSYCHOTHERAPY

Given the importance of touch in human development and the assumed role of physical contact in psychological homeostasis, why are there questions about the use of touch in psychotherapy? It would be logical to conclude that in psychotherapy, where an attempt is made to remedy problematic maturational experiences and problems in previous communications, touch may have a place. However, a litigious sociocultural context, in combination with sexual misconduct by some practitioners, has led toward a taboo of touch in psychotherapy. In order to understand the taboo, it is important to put the question of touch in psychotherapy in its historical context. (Smith raises many of these same points in Chapter 1.)

Although a taboo against sexual contact between healers and patients was established at least as long ago as the writings of Hippocrates (Perry, 1976), the taboo against touch between psychotherapists and patients is relatively new. Up until the advent of psychoanalysis in the late 1800s, psychiatry was largely the application of various physical interventions in an attempt to alter the minds of troubled individuals. These interventions frequently involved the use of touch and "laying on of hands" (Levitan & Johnson, 1986; Wilson, 1982).

In fact, touch was occasionally used in the early development of psychoanalysis in order to help patients express their emotions more easily. In his early work with hysteria, Freud used massage to the head and neck to facilitate catharsis of affect and hypnotic age regression in his patients. He and Breuer even allowed patients to touch them, as is clear from the early case studies (Breuer & Freud, 1895; Forer, 1969; Levitan & Johnson, 1986; Wilson, 1982). However, as Freud developed his work further, he gradually replaced the cathartic techniques with the analysis of transference and the technique of free association. Freud gradually recommended less "action" on the analyst's part, who was to remain a "blank slate" onto which the transference neurosis could be projected. In this context, touch was seen as a gratification of the patient's infantile needs and a contamination of the transference. The touch was thought to reify the relationship between analyst and patient, and thus to prevent the emergence of repressed unconscious content (Kupfermann & Smaldino, 1987). Another issue involved in Freud's objection to the use of touch rested on his fear that touch could stimulate sexual feelings in both analyst and patient—a response demonstrated in Freud's reaction to the "active technique" of Ferenczi (Ferenczi, 1953; Dupont, 1988). Ferenczi suggested that touch, including hugging and holding, could be useful as a way of repairing early damage in patients' experiences. Ferenczi also suggested other changes in technique, which he considered more important (Dupont, 1988), but it was the use of touch that deeply disturbed Freud and created a major rift between the two analysts. According to Jones (1955), Freud focused almost exclusively on a presumed erotic interpretation of the touch as the basis for his rejection of Ferenczi. Over time, the taboo against touch in psychoanalysis, and later in other psychodynamically oriented psychotherapies, became an entrenched dogma.

SEXUALIZED TOUCH IN PSYCHOTHERAPY

Beyond theoretical concerns, the inclusion of touch as an accepted tool in the psychotherapeutic repertoire can leave open the possibility for grave misuse. Certainly a number of arguments can be raised in opposition to the use of touch in psychotherapy, but none are more persuasive than the possibility of sexual acting out on the part of therapists. Without question, sexual activity with patients is a clear ethical, and in some areas legal, violation of great potential harm to patients (Brown, 1988; Delozier, 1994; Feldman-Summers & Jones, 1984; Sonne, Meyer, Borys, & Marshall, 1985; Sonne & Pope, 1991). Also without question, such acting out does occur.

Following a study of male physicians in the Los Angeles area, in which 59% of the respondents reported engaging in nonerotic hugging, kissing, and affectionate touching of patients (Kardener, Fuller, & Mensch, 1973), Holroyd and Brodsky (1977) conducted a similar study of both male and female doctoral-level psychotherapists. They found that approximately half of the respondents believed that nonerotic "hugging, kissing, or affectionate touching might be beneficial at least occasionally to both male and female patients" (p. 845). They also found that 34% of the therapists reported actually engaging in touch at least occasionally. Differences in the prevalence of touch were related to differences in theoretical orientation, with humanistic therapists using touch most often, and psychodynamic, behavioral, and rational/cognitive therapists touching least often.

Holroyd and Brodsky (1977) also found that in their sample, 5.5% of the male and 0.6% of the female therapists admitted having sexual intercourse with current patients. An additional 2.6% of the males and 0.3% of the females reported sexual intercourse with patients within 3 months of the termination of therapy. Of those who had intercourse with their patients, 80% repeated it. When all erotic contact with patients was considered, 10.9% of the males and 1.9% of the females reported such contact. These findings were very similar to the findings regarding sexual contact between female physicians and their patients (Perry, 1976), as well as the findings for the male physicians studied by Kardener et al. (1973). Holroyd and Brodsky (1980) published a follow-up report in which they reanalyzed their data in an attempt to discover a relationship between nonerotic and erotic touch. They found no general relationship, but found that therapists who touched patients of different genders differentially were at significantly higher risk for sexual contact with patients: Therapists who touched opposite-sex but not same-sex patients were much more likely to engage in sexual acting out. In other words, the therapists' own attitudes toward touch, whether erotic or nonerotic, were the key factors contributing to sexual misconduct.

Although these studies suggest that there is no relationship per se between nonerotic touch in psychotherapy and sexual acting out on the part of therapists, there are additional problems connected to an understanding of sexualized feelings in therapy. For example, there are gender differences in perceptions of touch. Abbey and Melby (1986) found that in general, men were more likely to perceive sexual intent in women, whereas women were less likely to perceive sexual intent in men, especially when the situation was ambiguous (e.g., casual touch, moderate interpersonal distance). On the other hand, men and women did not differ significantly in their evaluations of male therapists who touched their female patients (Suiter & Goodyear, 1985). Both groups saw the therapist who used the highest level of touch (semiembrace) as less trustworthy but more expert.

More importantly, there are difficulties in defining the boundary between nonerotic and erotic touching (Brodsky, 1985; Sponitz, 1972). It is possible that some of the findings of the limited number of studies of touch in psychotherapy may be contaminated by these problems in definition (see Alyn, 1988, and Willison & Masson, 1986, for a review). Brodsky (1985) has suggested that overt behavior is an insufficiently stringent ethical guideline. Instead, she suggests that "erotic touch" should be defined as any behavior that leads to sexual arousal on the part of either therapist or patient. In Brodsky's view, a therapist who continues to touch a patient after it becomes known that the touch is sexually arousing is engaging in deliberate sexual abuse.

It is important to note that the existence of sexual feelings in therapy is not uncommon. Pope, Keith-Spiegel, and Tabachnick (1986) noted that although 93.5% of their sample of psychologists never acted out sexually, only 13.2% reported never being sexually attracted to their patients. Male therapists were more likely to be attracted to patients than were female therapists, and younger therapists were more likely to be attracted to patients than were older therapists. In discussing this article, Hall (1987) noted that ethical education in psychotherapy programs is hampered by a failure to differentiate sexual feelings from sexual activity. However, when this differentiation is not made and sexual activity does occur, it is not at all clear that touch, in and of itself, is the culprit any more than other variables (e.g., personality dynamics of the perpetrating therapist).

INDICATIONS AND CONTRAINDICATIONS TO TOUCH

The evidence thus far available suggests that although sexual acting out does occur and that it is damaging when it does, there is little reason to assume that touch in psychotherapy is routinely sexualized, either in fact or in perception. But, beyond sexual acting out, there are other arguments regarding the use of touch in psychotherapy.

Most of these arguments center on the issue of "contamination of the transference" and a diminished motivation on the part of the patient in psychotherapy. Gutheil and Gabbard (1993) have gone so far as to state that all physical contact beyond a formal handshake is a boundary violation, and they are not alone in this view. Menninger (1958) declared that therapists who touch their patients are incompetent and criminal. These authorities and others have noted that physical contact places the therapist on the "slippery slope" toward inappropri-ate gratification of the needs of both patient and therapist, inevitably defeating the therapy.

Alyn (1988) has argued that touch between therapist and patient raises the issue of the power differential. She notes that it is more common for higher-status individuals to touch those of lower status, and that touch seldom occurs in the reverse direction. Because of this, she feels that a male therapist's touching a female patient is likely to contribute to a feeling of disempowerment in the woman, and that the touch is therefore potentially harmful for reasons unrelated to overt sexual misconduct.

However, many authors have taken a more moderate approach, stressing that touch may be used appropriately at times, but that there are clear contraindications as well. Mintz (1969), for example, stated that touch may be appropriately employed (1) as a form of symbolic parenting at those times when the patient is incapable of verbal interaction; (2) as a way of communicating acceptance when the patient's self-loathing is overwhelming; (3) as a means of strengthening or restoring reality contact; (4) as a means of controlled exploration of aggressive feelings (e.g., arm wrestling); and (5) as a natural expression of the therapist's feelings, provided that such expression is also a part of the overall therapeutic progression. Regarding this last point, Mintz noted that expressions of feeling are not necessarily appropriate even though they are authentic, and that touch should never be used when the feelings expressed are not authentic. Also, Mintz suggested that touch should never be used as a gratification of needs leading to avoidance of therapeutic material, or in instances in which the patient may be manipulating the therapist into supporting a position of helplessness.

Older (1982) suggested that touch can be used to (1) emphasize a verbal statement; (2) focus a patient's attention; and (3) reenergize a blocked patient. This last point echoes some recent arguments in favor of referring patients to massage therapists or other body workers when the therapy is blocked and the patient needs physical relaxation in order to contact sensations and feelings more effectively. Older also cited occasions when touch should be avoided: (1) when the therapist does not want to touch; (2) when the patient does not want to be touched; (3) when either the patient or the therapist believes the touch will not be helpful; or (4) when either therapist or patient feels manipulated by the touch. O'Hearne (1972) added that touch should be avoided when the patient is likely to misinterpret the touch (e.g., when he or she is overtly hostile or paranoid), or when the therapist is aware of harboring hostile feelings toward the patient.

THE CONTEXTS OF TOUCHING

It is tempting to assume simply that the appropriate application of touch can have a healing effect. Although this assumption awaits further exploration, we believe that the power and complexity of touch as a mode of communication requires a multifaceted analysis (Kertay & Reviere, 1993). For example, it is critical to place the use of touch in an ethical context that minimizes its potential abuses and maximizes its potential benefits. In order to make such an analysis, we believe that three related questions need to be addressed. First, what is appropriate in terms of touch? Second, how do we learn to recognize, in the course of a given therapy, an opening for appropriate touch? Third, how do we distinguish between such an opportunity and a time to withhold touch instead, perhaps relying on other means for processing the issues involved? We believe that the contexts surrounding the touch influence the answers to these questions by influencing the meaning assigned to the touch by both therapist and patient. Here, we briefly address some of the general considerations surrounding these questions; other chapters of this volume address more specific aspects.

We believe that it is important in discussing the application of touch to distinguish between the specifically body-oriented therapies, where touch is an intrinsic element of the therapy, and those therapies that are more verbally oriented. In the body-oriented therapies—such as bioenergetics, Reichian and neo-Reichian therapies, and "nonpsychological" therapies (e.g., Rolfing structural integration)—both therapist and patient expect touch to be a part of the process. In these therapies it is not a question of whether to touch, but rather of how to determine whether the patient is an appropriate candidate for the therapy, and how to process the feelings associated with the touch and body work. It is in the more traditionally verbal therapies that the decision to touch must be made, and the parameters of these decisions are complicated by the fact that touch is not presumed. In this chapter, we address ourselves primarily to the questions surrounding the use of touch in the verbal therapies, especially those that are psychodynamically oriented. We believe, however, that many of the same issues and concerns apply to body-oriented therapies, although they are applied in different ways.

Many contexts influence the perception of touch in the psychotherapeutic relationship. Of primary importance is the nature of the therapy relationship itself. Because of the dynamics of the therapist–patient relationship, the patient is likely to give a great deal of weight to the actions of the therapist. The therapist must be mindful of Alyn's (1988) admonition regarding power differentials and must carefully consider the impact of touch on the patient, as well as his or her own motivations in touching. When the therapist touches, the patient is "literally in the hands of the therapist," as Kepner (1987, p. 81) has stated, and it is critical that this contact be treated with the thoughtfulness it requires.

The Therapist's Context

The first context, then, consists of the therapist's own motivations, feelings, and thoughts in relation to touch. This context must be explored with the help of colleagues and supervisors before touch is used in the therapy relationship. A critical aspect of what makes a touch appropriate is that it is a genuine expression of the therapist's feelings, and, moreover, that it serves to further the growth of the patient rather than the needs of the therapist. In order for this condition to exist, the therapist must be cognizant of his or her own motivations in touching and must recognize his or her own needs. The therapist must be clear that the touch is not merely self-gratifying and must be able to maintain a focus on the needs of the patient. This means avoiding touch that is sexual, touch that is a subtle form of power or manipulation, and touch that is a means of "rescuing" the patient from his or her anxiety at those times when the therapist is perhaps even more uncomfortable than the patient. In general, this level of analysis requires that the therapist be exquisitely aware of countertransference responses, and that he or she be willing to monitor and process such responses internally and with trusted colleagues.

The Patient's Context

The second context influencing the interpretation of touch in a psychotherapy relationship involves the dynamics of the patient—that is, both diagnostic category or general level of functioning, and individual dynamics and issues. Goodman and Teicher (1988) have suggested a distinction based on whether the patient is "regressed" or "undeveloped." They suggest that a patient who is regressed is avoiding internal resources that can be brought to bear on a particular problem. They note that a regressed patient will be generally hampered by touch, and that the touch may serve to promote the regression by gratifying infantile needs in a manner that reifies the therapist as nurturer. In this case, the use of touch may impede the utilization and growth of ego functions that promote the ability for self-soothing and self-containment. On the other hand, an undeveloped or underdeveloped patient is one who is missing important aspects of social and emotional learning. Such a patient does not regress per se, but rather has deficits in internal resources. As such, the undeveloped patient is likely to be overwhelmed by his or her affect and is likely to be unable to negotiate the developmental process of the therapy without some type of support on the part of the therapist. For such a patient, touch may be used as a means of containing overwhelming affect, communicating safety, and providing a corrective experience for the nurturance that was insufficiently experienced during earlier development.

We believe that Goodman and Teicher's (1988) distinction can be useful and can be considered relative to familiar diagnostic categories or to theorized character structures in evaluating the use of touch with certain patterns of patient dynamics. For example, certain characterological structures, such as "hysterical" or "narcissistic" character organizations, can be considered predominantly "regressed." Other character structures, such as "schizoid" characters, can be considered predominantly "undeveloped." A therapist taking this approach would be more circumspect in evaluating the potential interpretations of touch in the hysterical patient, whereas he or she might consider the utility of touch with a patient with schizoid dynamics. However, it is our experience that few patients are fully one character "type" or another, and that the character types defined by these theorists tend to be reified, to the detriment of many patients. Even the most undeveloped patient has some resources on which to rely and may therefore experience regressions that may be harmfully gratified by certain forms of touch. Similarly, even the most "hysterical" patients have deficits in development that may be therapeutically treated through the containment and contact of appropriate touch. We believe, therefore, that Goodman and Teicher's (1988) distinction is best applied in a situation-specific manner. That is, in this patient at this time, will the touch serve to enhance internal resources? Or will it serve to circumvent internal resources and inappropriately distract the patient from the content of the therapy? Will the touch provide ego functions that can be internalized and utilized by the patient? Or will the touch collude with a desired infantile position that preempts the difficult but important use and growth of existing, if nascent, ego resources? Certain character structures may provide warning flags for the therapist to be circumspect, but the individual and his or her particular strengths and deficits will determine the appropriateness of the touch.

In considering the individual patient, therefore, the second contextual clue to the interpretation of the touch requires the therapist to ask whether touch will further therapy or collude to avoid it. If the touch is needed for containment of overwhelming affect, for guidance when verbal interaction is insufficient, or for contact when the patient feels overwhelmingly disconnected, then it may be useful as a human gesture that may communicate more effectively than words. If the touch gratifies a conscious or unconscious rescue fantasy, it is likely to delay the therapy at best and to derail it at worst. Even if satisfying for the moment, such touch can involve a collusion on the part of the therapist in keeping the patient dependent, potentially binding therapeutic progress.

The Therapeutic Alliance

The final context to be considered here is the nature and durability of the therapeutic alliance. If the therapeutic alliance is fragile, either because it is new or because of conflict between therapist and patient, touch is less likely to be helpful and more likely to be interpreted as aggressive or seductive. In general, we believe that touch must serve the conscious, agreed-upon goals and direction of the therapy as both explicitly contracted and implicitly communicated. Specifically, the therapist and patient must have a healthy working alliance, within which both parties make conscious decisions as to the nature of the therapeutic work. Furthermore, it is incumbent on the therapist to monitor this alliance and its fluctuations, as reflected in the vicissitudes of the deepening therapy relationship, in evaluating the utility of touch. In general, we suggest that touch is rarely helpful early in the therapy; that it is never helpful when it is routine and unconsidered; and that it is never appropriate when either the therapist or the patient is uncomfortable with touch. Although touch, such as a hug or a hand on the shoulder when the patient is severely distressed, can be helpful in building a therapeutic alliance by communicating support, we believe that such expressions should be thoughtfully considered and processed in the therapy. Such expressions are certainly human, but they can also serve to reduce anxiety prematurely and to set up an expectation on the part of the patient (or the therapist, for that matter) to avoid difficult therapeutic work through gratification, thus altering the intended direction or course of the therapeutic work. In addition, some patients may be frightened by touch early in the therapy, or they may experience its use outside the explicit contract for the therapy work as an intrusion.

It is of course possible to define the therapeutic alliance as involving touch from the outset, as is done in many of the "body-oriented" therapies and as we have noted above. However, even here, we believe it is critical to consider the contextual cues in deciding whether to accept the patient into such a therapy and in deciding when to begin body-oriented work. We believe that regressed, dependent patients with ill-defined ego boundaries are poor candidates for extensively touch-oriented therapies, especially in the early stages of the therapy. On the other hand, physically rigid and overdefended patients with good ego strength may be able to tolerate touch from the outset, whether the touch is from the therapist or from an adjunctive therapist to whom the main therapist refers the client. However, we know of therapists who have made healing, therapeutic interventions involving touch with just the types of patients for whom we urge caution, and we reiterate that this issue requires complex and thoughtful analysis.

GUIDELINES FOR THE CONSCIENTIOUS THERAPIST

As we have stated in our previous article (Kertay & Reviere, 1993), we believe that a rule- bound approach to questions surrounding touch is precluded by the complexities of the issues involved. Such decisions are best made on a case-by-case basis; the individual therapist, the unique patient and his or her dynamics, and the particular way the two interact must all be taken into consideration. However, we feel that guidelines can be offered for modification within the individual framework. In our 1993 article, we have proposed a three-level approach to decision making that considers the ethical, therapeutic, and theoretical issues involved.

Ethical Considerations

When a therapist is considering touch, the first level of consideration involves ethical issues. Some of the issues at this level are clear-cut and override individual contexts. When there is potential exploitation, whether sexual or based on a power differential, touch must be avoided. Sexual contact between therapist and patient is clearly inappropriate in any circumstance, and in any situation in which the possibility of sexual acting out is increased, touch should be avoided.

One of the major warning signs regarding potential exploitation is the tendency to touch patients on the basis of gender, as noted earlier. A therapist recognizing such a tendency is advised to stop all physical contact. Similarly, we agree with Brodsky's (1985) suggestion that overt behavior is an insufficiently stringent indicator of sexualized contact. Instead, sexual arousal on the part of either therapist or patient is an indication that all touch should be discontinued, and that the issues and feelings should be processed in the therapy and in supervision. Although we recognize that physical attraction between therapist and patient is not inherently problematic or unusual, we argue that sexual arousal and touch should not occur simultaneously in the therapy. When they do, an unclear boundary is created, and the safety of the relationship is compromised.

It is also important to note that exploitation of the patient can occur without overt sexual themes; it may occur whenever the touch gratifies the therapist's needs at the expense of the patient. Following Alyn's (1988) argument, we believe it is especially critical for male therapists who touch female patients to be mindful of the potential for subtle forms of coercion based on a power differential.

Beyond such relatively clear-cut ethical concerns, the therapist who is considering whether or not to touch within the psychotherapy relationship is advised to be prepared to process the attendant issues throughout the therapy. The therapist is advised to consider carefully the meanings of touch, both positive and negative, in his or her own life. What are the therapist's motivations for touch, and how can he or she be clear about the countertransferential feelings associated with the use of touch? These questions apply to the question of touch in general, as well as to work with a specific patient. We advise the therapist to be in individual or group supervision that addresses the use of touch specifically and in which the therapist is free to discuss the nature of personal thoughts and feelings associated with touch.

Therapeutic Considerations

The psychotherapist who is considering touch with a specific patient is also advised to consider carefully the needs of the particular patient and the aims of therapy. Geib's (1982) guidelines are useful in this context. To reiterate: Touch is most likely to be helpful and appropriate (1) when the touch is congruent with the experienced level of intimacy in the therapeutic relationship; (2) when it is congruent with the patient's perceived needs; and (3) when both patient and therapist are open to discussing the touch and attendant feelings. The conscientious therapist might ask these questions: Does the patient wish to be touched, and in what way are these wishes being communicated? What is the nature of the transference, and in what way does the therapist respond to the transference? What is the patient's history with touch, and how free is the patient in discussing his or her feelings in relation to the therapist?

In particular, therapists may find themselves touching on the basis of a need to feel "helpful" when a patient is distressed. Although this is not necessarily problematic, often a therapist seeks to soothe a patient physically when in fact the patient needs to tolerate and explore the pain being experienced. In any of these circumstances, the touch should be carefully considered, discontinued when it is believed to interfere with the patient's progress, and processed in the therapy and in supervision.

We believe that severely regressed, poorly boundaried patients are in general poor candidates for being touched, at least early in the therapy. However, as we have noted above, even such distinctions are secondary to consideration of the particular case and the particular skills and training of the therapist.

Theoretical Issues: Communicating with Touch and Listening for Feedback

The psychotherapist who has decided to touch, based on personal ethical preparation and a careful consideration of the therapeutic relationship, is further advised to consider two theoretical aspects of the touch itself. The first aspect of a touch communication is assertive and expressive; that is, the touch is intended to convey some meaning through the contact. This aspect of the touch involves "doing something" with the patient. The second aspect of a touch communication is reserved and receptive; that is, the touch conveys information back to the therapist in some form of feedback. This aspect of the touch involves "listening" to the patient's response to the touch, as well as monitoring the therapist's own reactions.

Before beginning touch, the therapist is advised to discuss the issue of touch with the patient in a matter-of-fact manner. The patient should be asked to discuss his or her history with touch, feelings related to the therapist's touching, and fantasies and fears when touch is imagined. The parameters of the intended touch should be discussed, including a clear statement of safety with regard to sexual boundaries. Although it is not practical to discuss in advance each incidence of future touch, the therapist is advised to announce verbally the intent to touch, or to ask for the patient's permission to touch, and to give the patient the opportunity to decline such touch. Ideally, this verbalization should occur prior to each occurrence of touch.

In relation to the active aspect of the touch, the therapist is advised to consider the intended meaning of the touch. We believe that appropriate uses of touch include the communication of containment for overwhelming affect, reassurance for the patient who feels disconnected, and soothing of childlike ego states overwhelmed by the current situation of the therapy. The therapist is strongly advised to avoid touch that deflates rather than enhances the internal resources of the patient, as well as touch that might be experienced as aggressive and/or seductive.

In relation to the receptive aspect of the touch, the conscientious

BRYAN COLLEGE LIBRARY

therapist attends to the responses of the patient, both verbal and nonverbal. How does the patient respond to being touched? What meaning does the patient assign to the touch? How is the touch received on both feeling and interpretive bases? Both positive and negative responses should be noted and processed, providing a verbal context for the touch. In addition, the conscientious therapist similarly monitors his or her own countertransferential responses to touching, as noted above. Is the therapist aware of feeling manipulated into touching, or aware of wanting to manipulate the patient? Does the touch feel like a genuine expression of contact, or does it feel like a token activity devoid of feeling? Such responses are useful indicators of the perceived meaning in the touch and become important material for discussion in the therapy.

Finally, once a decision is made to utilize touch, it is most helpful if that intervention can be processed directly in the therapy. This processing occurs as soon after the touch as is practical, especially if the touch has been noted to arouse sexual, aggressive, or otherwise uncomfortable feelings in either the patient or the therapist. However, even if the touch is apparently experienced as a positive communication, the patient should be given the opportunity to state the nature of his or her experience. Responses noted by the therapist during the touch should be offered to the patient verbally, and the nature of the affective, physical, and cognitive associations should be explored.

The importance of processing the feelings brought up by touch in psychotherapy is highlighted in the only published study of patients' experiences of touch to date. Horton, Clance, Sterk-Elifson, and Emshoff (1995) presented a study of 231 patients who reported significant experiences of touch in psychotherapy. The study provided evidence for the existence of positive interpretations of touch; the relatively rare sexualized interpretations of touch; and Geib's (1982) suggestion that patients are most likely to have positive experiences of touch when the touch is perceived to be congruent with the level of intimacy in the relationship as well as congruent with their own needs, and when both patient and therapist are open to discussing the feelings that arise in response to the touch. (This study is discussed in more detail by Horton in Chapter 9 of this volume.)

CONCLUSIONS

Although we recognize that it would be easier simply to "outlaw" touch in psychotherapy or otherwise create rules to regulate it, we believe this mode of communication to be too powerful and too complex to lend itself to simplistic conclusions. Furthermore, such an approach can dehumanize therapy by artificially removing or strictly regulating a very natural form of human communication. However, we do not recommend a carte blanche approach to touch. Instead, we suggest that touch may have a place in psychotherapy, but that its application requires careful thought, in-depth understanding of the therapist's own motivations, and a careful consideration based on the needs of the patient. Such an approach assumes that the therapist is willing to make the considerable effort to process his or her own feelings, alone and in consultation with colleagues and supervisors who are skilled in the application of touch. The therapist who is unwilling to make this effort is indeed in danger of finding himself or herself on the "slippery slope" leading to personal difficulty and potential abuse of the patient. We acknowledge that our proffered suggestions are a bare skeleton to guide the conscientious psychotherapist; nevertheless, we hope that they provide a framework for the decision-making process involved before, during, and after the decision to touch is made.

ACKNOWLEDGMENT

Parts of this chapter are loosely based on Kertay and Reviere (1993).

REFERENCES

Abbey, A., & Melby, C. (1986). The effects of nonverbal cues on gender differences in perceptions of sexual intent. *Sex Roles, 15,* 283–298.

Alyn, J. H. (1988). The politics of touch in therapy: A response to Willison and Masson. *Journal of Counseling and Development, 66,* 432–433.

Breuer, J., & Freud, S. (1895). *Studien über hysterie.* Leipzig: Franz Deuticke.

Brodsky, A. M. (1985). Sex between therapists and patients: Ethical gray areas. *Psychotherapy in Private Practice, 3*(1), 57–62.

Brown, L. (1988). Harmful effects of post-termination sexual and romantic relationships with former clients. *Psychotherapy, 25,* 249–255.

Bushnell, E. W., & Boudreau, J. P. (1993). Motor development and the mind: The potential role of motor abilities as a determinant of aspects of perceptual development. *Child Development, 64,* 1005–1021.

Delozier, P. P. (1994). Therapist sexual misconduct. *Women and Therapy, 15,* 55–67.

Dubovsky, S. L., & Groban, S. E. (1975). Congenital absence of sensation. *Psychoanalytic Study of the Child, 30,* 49–73.

Dupont, J. (Ed.). (1988). *The clinical diary of Sandor Ferenczi.* Cambridge, MA: Harvard University Press.

Feldman-Summers, S., & Jones, G. (1984). Psychological impacts of sexual contact between therapists or other health care professionals and their clients. *Journal of Consulting and Clinical Psychology, 52,* 1054–1061.

Ferenczi, S. (1953). *The theory and technique of psychoanalysis.* New York: Basic Books.

Fisher, S. (1970). *Body experience in fantasy and behavior.* New York: Appleton-Century-Crofts.

Fisher, S. (1986). *Development and structure of the body image* (2 vols.). Hillsdale, NJ: Erlbaum.

Fisher, S. (1990). The evolution of psychological concepts about the body. In T. F. Cash & T. Pruzinsky (Eds.), *Body images: Development, deviance, and change.* New York: Guilford Press.

Fisher, S., & Cleveland, S. E. (1968). *Body image and personality* (rev. ed.). New York: Dover.

Forer, B. R. (1969). The taboo against touching in psychotherapy. *Psychotherapy: Theory, Research, and Practice, 6*(4), 229–231.

Geib, P. G. (1982). The experience of nonerotic physical contact in traditional psychotherapy: A critical investigation of the taboo against touch. *Dissertation Abstracts International, 43,* 1–13A.

Goodman, M., & Teicher, A. (1988). To touch or not to touch. *Psychotherapy, 25,* 492–500.

Grunau, R. V., Whitfield, M. F., Petrie, J. H., & Fryer, E. L. (1994). Early pain experience, child factors, and family factors as precursors of somatization: A prospective study of extremely premature and fullterm children. *Pain, 56,* 353–359.

Gupta, M. A., & Schork, N. J. (1995). Touch deprivation has an adverse effect on body image: Some preliminary observations. *International Journal of Eating Disorders, 17,* 185–189.

Gutheil, T., & Gabbard, G. (1993). The concept of boundaries in clinical practice: Theoretical and risk-management dimensions. *American Journal of Psychiatry, 150,* 188–196.

Hall, J. E. (1987). Gender-related ethical dilemmas and ethics education. *Professional Psychology: Research and Practice, 18,* 573–579.

Harlow, H. F. (1958). The nature of love. *American Psychologist, 13,* 673–685.

Holroyd, J. C., & Brodsky, A. (1977). Psychologists' attitudes and practices regarding erotic and nonerotic physical contact with patients. *American Psychologist, 32,* 839–843.

Holroyd, J. C., & Brodsky, A. (1980). Does touching patients lead to sexual intercourse? *Professional Psychology, 11,* 807–811.

Horner, A. J. (1984). *Object relations and the developing ego in therapy.* Northvale, NJ: Jason Aronson.

Horner, A. J. (1990). *The primacy of structure: Psychotherapy of underlying character pathology.* Northvale, NJ: Jason Aronson.

Horton, J. A., Clance, P. R., Sterk-Elifson, C., & Emshoff, J. (1995). Touch in psychotherapy: A survey of patients' experiences. *Psychotherapy, 32,* 443–457.

Jones, E. (1955). *The life and work of Sigmund Freud: Vol. 2. Years of maturity.* New York: Basic Books.

Kardener, S. H., Fuller, M., & Mensh, I. N. (1973). A survey of physicians' attitudes and practices regarding erotic and nonerotic contact with patients. *American Journal of Psychiatry, 130,* 1077–1081.

Kepner, J. I. (1987). *Body process: A Gestalt approach to working with the body in psychotherapy.* New York: Gestalt Institute of Cleveland Press.

Kernberg, O. F. (1975). *Borderline conditions and pathological narcissism.* Northvale, NJ: Jason Aronson.

Kernberg, O. F. (1976). *Object relations theory and clinical psychoanalysis.* Northvale, NJ: Jason Aronson.

Kertay, L., & Reviere, S. L. (1993). The use of touch in psychotherapy: Theoretical and ethical considerations. *Psychotherapy, 30,* 32–40.

Kohut, H. (1971). *The analysis of the self.* New York: International Universities Press.

Kreuger, D. (1989). *Body self and psychological self: Developmental and clinical integration in disorders of the self.* New York: Brunner/Mazel.

Kreuger, D. (1990). Developmental and psychodynamic perspectives on body-image change. In T. F. Cash & T. Pruzinsky (Eds.), *Body images: Development, deviance, and change.* New York: Guilford Press.

Kupfermann, K., & Smaldino, C. (1987). The vitalizing and revitalizing experience of reliability: The place of touch in psychotherapy. *Clinical Social Work Journal, 15*(3), 223–235.

Levitan, A. A., & Johnson, J. M. (1986). The role of touch in healing and hypnotherapy. *American Journal of Clinical Hypnosis, 28*(4), 218–223.

Mahler, M. S. (1968). *On human symbiosis and the vicissitudes of individuation.* New York: International Universities Press.

Mahler, M. S., & McDevitt, J. B. (1982). Thoughts on the emergence of the sense of self, with particular emphasis on the body self. *Journal of the American Psychoanalytic Association, 30,* 919–937.

Mahler, M. S., Pine, F., & Bergman, A. (1975). *The psychological birth of the human infant: Symbiosis and individuation.* New York: Basic Books.

Masters, R. (1987). The psyche and the skin. *Neurologic Clinics, 5*(3), 483–497.

Menninger, K. (1958). *Theory of psychoanalytic technique.* New York: Basic Books.

Mintz, E. E. (1969). On the rationale of touch in psychotherapy. *Psychotherapy: Theory, Research, and Practice, 6*(4), 232–234.

Montagu, A. (1971). *Touching: The human significance of the skin.* New York: Columbia University Press.

O'Hearne, J. J. (1972). How can we reach patients most effectively? *International Journal of Group Psychotherapy, 22,* 446–454.

Older, J. (1982). *Touching is healing.* New York: Stein & Day.

Perry, J. A. (1976). Physicians' erotic and nonerotic physical involvement with patients. *American Journal of Psychiatry, 133,* 838–848.

Pope, K. S., Keith-Spiegel, P., & Tabachnick, B. G. (1986). Sexual attraction to clients: The human therapist and the (sometimes) inhuman training system. *American Psychologist, 41,* 147–158.

Schilder, P. (1935). *The image and appearance of the human body.* New York: International Universities Press.

Shontz, F. C. (1974). Body image and its disorders. *International Journal of Psychiatry in Medicine, 5,* 461–471.

Shontz, F. C. (1975). *The psychological aspects of physical illness and disability.* New York: Macmillan.

Shontz, F. C. (1990). Body image and physical disability. In T. F. Cash & T. Pruzinsky (Eds.), *Body images: Development, deviance, and change.* New York: Guilford Press.

Sivik, T. (1993). Alexithymia and hypersensitivity to touch and palpation. *Integrative Physiological and Behavioral Science, 28,* 130–136.

Sonne, J., Meyer, C. B., Borys, D., & Marshall, V. (1985). Clients' reactions to sexual intimacy in therapy. *American Journal of Orthopsychiatry, 55,* 183–189.

Sonne, J., & Pope, K. (1991). Treating victims of therapist–patient sexual involvement. *Psychotherapy, 28,* 174–187.

Spitz, R. A. (1945). An inquiry into the genesis of psychiatric conditions in early childhood. *Psychoanalytic Study of the Child, 1,* 53–74.

Sponitz, H. (1972). Touch countertransference in group psychotherapy. *International Journal of Group Psychotherapy, 22,* 455–463.

Suiter, R. L., & Goodyear, R. K. (1985). Male and female counselor and client perceptions of four levels of counselor touch. *Journal of Counseling Psychology, 32,* 645–648.

Willison, B. G., & Masson, R. L. (1986). The role of touch in therapy: An adjunct to communication. *Journal of Counseling and Development, 64,* 497–500.

Wilson, J. M. (1982). The value of touch in psychotherapy. *American Journal of Orthopsychiatry, 52*(1), 65–72.

Winnicott, D. W. (1965). *The maturational processes and the facilitating environment.* New York: International Universities Press.

3

A TAXONOMY AND ETHICS OF TOUCH IN PSYCHOTHERAPY

Edward W. L. Smith

"A rose is a rose is a rose," Gertrude Stein told us. But to play off her famous line, I say, "A touch is not a touch is not a touch." Touch appears in a great variety of nuances, forms, and intentions. Nevertheless, too many mavens of psychotherapy ethics speak as if "touch" is a homogeneous, unidimensional phenomenon in all its contexts and occurrences. We find examples of argument for or against "touch," often without clear definition of how, when, by whom, under what conditions, and for what purpose "touch" is used. I maintain that it is only through taking account of such parameters that we can come to meaningful ethics of touch in psychotherapy.

In order to identify types of touch that may occur in psychotherapy, I offer the following taxonomy. First, let us define those forms of touch that are now taboo. By so doing, perhaps we can clear ground for a discussion of the other forms of touch that may or may not be ethical; decisions about these forms require a very careful consideration of the above-mentioned parameters.

TABOO FORMS OF TOUCH

The first major taboo pertains to sexual touching. The code of ethics of the American Psychological Association (1992) states baldly, "Psychologists do not engage in sexual intimacies with current patients or clients" (p. 1605). This ethical proclamation has become the standard and has been taken as a model by other mental health professions. In addition, several states have recently passed laws making therapist–client sexual contact a punishable offense. Thus, sexual touching is clearly taboo.

One of my early supervisors, John Warkentin, codeveloper of experiential psychotherapy at the Atlanta Psychiatric Clinic, stated clearly that therapy doesn't work when the therapist touches with erotic interest. Building on this teaching, I wrote in one chapter of *The Body in Psychotherapy:* "That is not ethically guided work when the therapist touches in order to get turned on. The reason for touching must be nonerotic, nonseductive. Again, the patient is not here for the therapist's entertainment, erotic or otherwise. The therapist's touch must be respectful of the patient's therapeutic need" (Smith, 1985, p. 150).

Moreover, the bulk of reported evidence suggests that more often than not, the client suffers when sexual touching occurs in psychotherapy. And, again, professional ethics (and the laws of several states) now clearly prohibit this kind of touching. When one joins a helping profession, one is given privileges, but at the same time one incurs obligations. The ethical code is a major and serious obligation.

The second taboo concerning touch in psychotherapy pertains to hostile or aggressive touch. This taboo is so self-evident as to be easily overlooked. Obviously, physical attack on a client is unjustifiable. But in this instance it behooves us not to be blinded too easily by an obvious, black-and-white statement. Some years ago a therapist friend of mine was attacked and beaten during a therapy session. More recently, literature has appeared documenting the physical dangers of being a therapist (Travers, 1994, 1995). If a therapist is physically attacked by a client, would any reasonable person object that the therapist was unethical for defending himself or herself? Surely not. If this is so, then we cannot in complete accuracy say simply that it is unethical to aggress physically against a client. We must qualify the ethical principle to take particular circumstances into consideration. I take my lead here from the code of ethics of aikido (Westbrook & Ratti, 1970). As a martial art having no offensive moves, but focusing exclusively on defense, aikido is highly sensitive to ethical nuances. Four ethical levels are recognized in defense in combat. The lowest ethical level is unprovoked aggression in the form of direct attack. The second lowest level is to provoke an attack from another and then act in self-defense. At the third level one neither attacks nor provokes attack, but uses undue force in defending oneself, resulting in an unnecessary degree of injury to one's attacker. The fourth level is the ultimate goal in ethical self-defense. At this level one defends against unprovoked attack, using only the force necessary to neutralize the attack. The ideal is to stop the attacker while minimizing harm to him or her. Self-defense, ethically conducted, is itself considered of ethical value. By neutralizing an unprovoked attacker, one not only saves oneself from pain and injury, but saves the attacker from the karma of having inflicted unprovoked injury.

In therapy, then, the ethical commandment is not to act out unprovoked aggression and not to provoke aggression as an excuse to aggress against the client in "self-defense." This much, I believe, is obvious and serves as the basis of the taboo against physical aggression toward clients. We must, however, admit the existence of a gray zone, in which there is occasion for self-defense in the face of unprovoked attack. Skill at self-defense thus emerges as a factor to consider. In a case of alleged self-defense, did the therapist neutralize the client's attack, or did he or she go beyond this (or perhaps even intend to harm)?

FIVE FORMS OF TOUCH NOT EXPLICITLY TABOO

I turn now to the nontaboo and therefore more controversial areas of touch, where we may expect gray zones and murkiness to be the rule. Crystal clarity and simplicity are not to be found here. So, to continue the taxonomy, I add "inadvertent touch." By this term, I mean touching that is not intentional—bumping into or brushing up against another while gesturing or moving about. Taken at face value, such touches are accidental, the products of inattention or incoordination. Graceless as they may be, at least on the social level they are usually passed off with no more than an "Excuse me." If, on the other hand, one wishes to depart the social level and wax psychodynamic, then even an inadvertent touch must be examined for the unconscious motive or meaning underlying it. It is precisely this motive or meaning that is then the focus of the ethical question. Whether it is accidental or a thinly disguised manifestation of an unconscious urge, inadvertent touch must be acknowledged as a category of touch that can occur in the psychotherapy setting.

Inadvertent touch is not intentional, at least consciously. However, there may be touch that is intentional but made to look inadvertent. The purpose may be taboo touch, such as in frottage, where the intention is sexual touch made to appear accidental. Or it may be a hostile touch made to seem accidental, such as bumping forcefully into another person or stepping on his or her foot. I mention the example of stepping on another's foot here to indicate the range of possible motives, from an area of ethical taboo (hostile/aggressive intent) to an area of psychotherapeutic benefit. I refer to one of the myriad stories told of Milton Erickson, which may or may not be apocryphal. As I heard the story, Erickson treated a young girl who would not leave her house because she was so ashamed of her feet, which she perceived as too big. Responding to her mother's request, Erickson went to the girl's home and chatted with her for a while, never mentioning his real purpose for being there. As he was leaving, he stepped on one of the girl's feet and muttered something like "If you'd grow those things large enough, this wouldn't happen." As the story goes, the girl relinquished her distorted body image and was able to leave the house in relative comfort. The point for us here is that this apparently inadvertent touch was not so at all, but was a very intentional touch with therapeutic aim. In the scheme of the taxonomy that I am presenting, this was a touch expressive of the therapeutic relationship, disguised as inadvertent touch. Such a maneuver was, of course, congruent with Erickson's indirect therapeutic style.

Another category of touch is the "conversational marker." Such touch is used as physical punctuation for one's conversation. To get or maintain someone's attention or to emphasize a point, one may touch a hand, a knee, or a shoulder.

Yet another type of touch in the taxonomy is "socially stereotyped touch." These are highly ritualized touches that carry a consensual meaning within a culture or a subculture. They are similar in nature to pantomime gestures, differing in that they involve physical contact. The handshake and the greeting embrace are examples of socially stereotyped touch.

There also occurs "touch as expression of the therapeutic relationship." If, for example, a therapy relationship is such that the therapist gives comfort when the client is grieving, then the therapist may put an arm around the client's shoulder. Or, if a therapist is engaged in a regressive, reparenting mode of therapy, he or she may hold the client like a child. This category of touch includes, then, holding, rocking, embracing, hand holding, and all such parental, "big brother," "big sister," and "buddy" kinds of touch.

Finally, to complete the taxonomy, there is "touch as technique." By this, I mean the technical use of touch as is found in Reichian orgonomy, bioenergetics, core energetics, radix, Pesso–Boyden system psychomotor (PBSP) therapy, organismic psychotherapy, Hakomi, and related systems. What characterizes these technical uses of touch is a clearly defined manner of touch with a prescribed use. How to touch, where on the client's body to touch, and (in some cases) for how long to touch are all prescribed for particular therapeutic purposes. (For an extensive study of these body-oriented systems of psychotherapy and their techniques, I refer the reader to *The Body in Psychotherapy* [Smith, 1985], as well as to Chapter 1 of the present volume.)

To summarize the discussion thus far, there are many forms of touch, arising for different purposes and from different motives. Any meaningful discussion of the ethics of touch in psychotherapy must first define the type of touch. For, as I have suggested, "A touch is not a touch is not a touch." (See Table 3.1.)

FACTORS INFLUENCING THE NUANCED MEANINGS OF TOUCH

Having established the need for a taxonomy of touch and having offered such a taxonomy, I come now to three basic and highly important considerations. The first, a basic axiom of communication theory, is that the message sent is not necessarily the message received. A few moments' reflection surely verifies this. So the therapist may touch with a particular intention (or without intention, in the case of inadvertent touch), but in interpreting that touch the client may be more or less accurate as to its intended meaning. It is important, therefore, that the therapist be alert to the possibility of misunderstanding and be quick to recognize it when it occurs, so that it can then be addressed and (ideally) resolved. With certain types of touch, such as a technical touch, an explanation of procedure and intention beforehand may be advisable. The same is true with more emotionally intimate touch, such as holding. This explanation is especially important before a relationship of trust has been established, as in the case of new clients and those clients whose character structure makes trust

TABLE 3.1. Taxonomy of Touch in Psychotherapy

Considered acceptable or unacceptable (depending on circumstances)
Inadvertent touch
Conversational markers
Socially stereotyped touch
Touch as an expression of the therapeutic relationship
Technical touch
Taboo
Hostile/aggressive touch (does not include self-defense that neutralizes a client's attack)
Sexual touch

an ongoing issue. I return later to this topic of explaining touch to the client.

The second consideration involves what anthropologists have identified as "cultural relativity." That is, the meaning of a behavior can be understood only in relation to the culture in which it occurs. Thus, a given behavior may have one meaning in one culture but quite a different meaning in another. Furthermore, cultural relativity applies even to what may be identified as subcultures. Cultural relativity may be a further cause for the above-mentioned axiom that the message received may not be the message sent. As a carrier of meaning, intended or not, touch shows a high degree of cultural relativity.

Closely related to touch is the use of physical space in communicating. Such proxemic behavior has been studied cross-culturally and has proven to be, as might well be expected, highly relative to the culture in which it occurs (Hall, 1973). Of particular importance to psychotherapy is the fact that individuals tend to define an area around them as "personal space," and that the distance included in personal space differs from culture to culture. If someone moves into this personal space without invitation, the person thus approached may feel crowded or intruded upon. We speak of "having our space invaded." The impact of coming into someone's personal space differs only by degree from a physical touch, and therefore requires the same consideration. A problem may arise if the therapist and client do not share the same cultural or personal proxemic norm. A therapist may be experienced as "distant," "respectful," or "invasive" without feeling or intending to be so, if he or she does not understand the rules governing personal space in the client's culture or subculture. Clearly, any therapist who works with clients of diverse cultures or even subcultures must learn the norms for proxemic as well as for touching behavior.

As a third consideration, I want to emphasize that communication through touch is in general more emotionally powerful than verbal communication, and at the same time is more ambiguous. Thus, touch is both powerful and risky. The therapist who touches may make stronger statements of presence and more forceful therapeutic interventions than the therapist who limits himself or herself to the verbal. In so doing, however, the therapist who touches introduces more potential for ambiguity, and thereby a greater possibility of misunderstanding.

These, then, are three considerations fundamental to the understanding of the ethics of touch in psychotherapy. To reiterate, the message sent is not necessarily the message received; the meaning of touch is culturally relative; and touch is often emotionally more powerful than verbal communication, while also being more ambiguous.

DECIDING WHEN AND WHEN NOT TO TOUCH

The central question that emerges in the wake of the discussion thus far is the question of when to touch. In the service of attempting to elucidate such a murky question, I am going to introduce a 2 × 2 decision table (see Table 3.2). The table includes two dimensions: a "theory" dimension and an "ethics" dimension. Previous discussions of touch in psychotherapy have sometimes failed to differentiate these two dimensions, thereby confusing the question. These two dimensions are distinct, but interact in the making of an ethical decision concerning touch, as we shall see.

Theoretical Considerations

On the theory dimension, the question is whether the theoretical base that guides one's therapeutic work supports the use of touch or not. By "theory," I mean the conceptual system out of which one operates—the more or less organized set of guiding principles that one uses in planning, executing, and justifying the conduct of psychotherapy. So one's "theory" may be a school of therapy, an eclectic combination of schools, or (to use an increasingly preferred term) an integrative approach. Depending on the school or component schools, the theory may be more or less data-driven. That is to say, some therapeutic approaches enjoy greater support from empirical research than others. Thus, within the term "theory" I include the range of positions from pure theory, through theory guided by clinical experience or anecdote, to theory closely allied to careful research, to "atheoretical" techniques (those that have support from research or clinical experience but are not understood through a larger theoretical frame).

One's theory may allow or may not allow for physical contact in general. Or it may offer a rule or guideline that can be applied in a specific, concrete therapeutic situation. For example, orthodox psychoanalysis would say "No" to touch as technique, touch as expression of therapeutic relationship, and touch as conversational marker; it would

TABLE 3.2. Decision Table for Each Kind and Instance of Touch

		Ethics	
		Yes	No
Theory	Yes		
	No		

perhaps say "No" to socially stereotyped touch; and it would probably regard inadvertent touch as highly suspicious, pending its analysis with a supervisor. The practitioner of such a theoretical approach is guided, then, not to touch at all, or to do so only with great caution and restriction (e.g., a handshake). If one's theory predicts that physical contact will interfere with the optimal development of the transference, then one should avoid touching a client. If touching is seen theoretically as possibly fulfilling an infantile wish, and in turn shifting focus from the analysis of that wish, then the analyst will not want to give nurturing touch.

I find another example of a generalized prohibition of touch in an article that takes a political (theoretical) stance:

> The predominant therapy situation of male therapist and female client replicates the prevailing power dynamics of the culture. Although nonerotic touch may not be unethical, it may very well reinforce the already unequal power relationship between therapist and client. . . . It may also reproduce conditions in which the client's aspirations, achievements, or hopes are devalued. In these ways, counselor touch may very well inhibit the client's development of self-esteem, autonomy, and ultimately, an effective resolution of the conflicts for which she or he sought help. (Alyn, 1988, p. 433)

Theoretical guidelines are sometimes offered with greater subtlety, avoiding the absolutist position never to touch. A prime example is the following:

> Physical touch as a part of psychodynamic psychotherapy is appropriate and useful under very limited circumstances. The decision is to be based on a careful evaluation of the state of the patient. The patient who is regressed is most likely to experience the touch as an encouragement toward continued regression and dependency. The nondeveloped patient, who has not matured to the point of adequate and acceptable functioning, may well profit from judicious and finely tuned physical touch experiences. (Goodman & Teicher, 1988, p. 492)

In a paper originally presented at a psychoanalytic meeting, the following cautious use of touching as a procedure was suggested:

> A particular psychotherapeutic procedure described by the authors as "The Revitalizing Experience of Reliability," is used as an adjunct to enhance the effectiveness of treatment. Characteristically, it is a nonmanipulative, nonseductive procedure used during particular stressful times with certain patients—adults as well as children—to facilitate a

confirmation of the self as separate from others. It should also instill in the patient a feeling of increased safety and reliability as well as promoting basic trust in self and others with the ultimate goal of reintegration of a fragmented ego. Such an adjunct can take various forms. The one described here is a highly controversial one, physical touch. (Kupfermann & Smaldino, 1987, p. 223)

In these three examples, then, we find a theoretical position of "No" or a theoretical position advocating very cautious and judicious use of touch under clearly defined circumstances, taking into consideration the characterological level of the client.

Viewing touch with perhaps less caution and less as an "adjunctive procedure" than is true in the examples above, certain regressive therapies and humanistic therapies are inclined to a "Yes." They see touch as a core and vital dimension of the expression of the therapeutic relationship, or at least as an acceptable aspect of this expression. Holding and touching are seen as avenues for the authentic expression of caring, concern, affection, and presence, thus providing an emotionally corrective experience for the client.

By definition, those schools of therapy that use touch techniques would vote "Yes" to touch on theoretical grounds. In any specific therapeutic situation, the question of whether or not to touch is expanded into the question of which of the myriad techniques is most appropriate, if any.

In the decision model that I am introducing, the theoretical consideration of whether or not to touch is critical. In the absence of catholicity in the field of psychotherapy, one is left to pick and choose from the array of therapies and techniques available. Once one is committed to a theoretical stance, that position may prohibit one from touching in general or under certain defined circumstances. Lacking such an interdiction, one then has to make the ethical decision per se. It is this dimension of the decision table to which I now turn.

Ethical Considerations

The ethical choice of "Yes" to touch, as I view it, involves three considerations. The first is a question of adequate theoretical/technical training. That is to say, has the therapist had sufficient education to comprehend the theory well enough to be guided by it? Does he or she understand the theory's range of applicability and its degree of certainty, born of research validation (if available)? Does he or she know the evaluative signs and indications, and the rules that allow the bridging of theory and praxis? And has the therapist had adequate supervision in the use of the methods and techniques to employ them competently? An affirmative answer to these and related questions is requisite to an ethical "Yes" in the decision table.

The second consideration is what I have called the "ego-syntonic imperative" (Smith, 1985, 1992):

> By this term I mean that for one to function optimally in the therapeutic role it is essential that he or she relate to the patient only in ways that are congruent with who that therapist is. . . . So, if a therapist feels like herself or himself in using a technique, if that technique seems to flow out of her or him, then it is an appropriate technique to keep in one's repertoire. Another facet of the ego-syntonic imperative is that the patient must work in the therapist's way, a way which allows the therapist to keep her or his integrity. . . . If the patient wants some other kind of work, something which I don't do, then it is better not to see that patient. As Barry Stevens (1970, p. 7) put it, "When the wrong man uses the right means, the right means work in the wrong way." (Smith, 1985, p. 148)

The client's need is the third consideration. Touching, in any of its intentional forms, should be done when, in the therapist's considered opinion, it is in the service of the therapeutic need of the client.

In the decision table, therefore, a "Yes" is appropriate on the ethical dimension when these three criteria are met: The therapist is adequately trained, theoretically and technically; the touch is ego-syntonic for the therapist; and, in the therapist's best judgment, the touch is congruent with the client's therapeutic need. When these three criteria are not met, then obviously the ethical decision concerning touch is "No." If the therapist's training has not included touch, or if the training has been inadequate in terms of either theory or supervised practice, then it is incumbent upon the therapist not to use therapeutic touch. If touching is ego-dystonic for the therapist, the ethical decision for the therapist is "No." And if the touch would be based on a personal need of the therapist, the ethical decision is "No."

When Not to Touch: Guidance from Hindu Psychology

This last statement invites expatiation. In understanding the personal needs of the therapist, I have found the *chakra* model, taken from Hindu psychology, to be most useful. This is a highly complex model, so I will give only a brief overview of the aspects of it that are most apropos. (For a more thorough discussion, with clinical application, I refer the reader to my chapter "Anahata, Freeze-Dried" [Smith, 1994].)

The seven *chakras* represent levels of consciousness. Figuratively located along the spine and at the throat and head, they symbolize the raising of consciousness from lower levels to upper, spiritual levels. Each may be thought of as a template through which one's experience is filtered. So, as an event occurs, one experiences that event in a manner guided by the selectivity and sensitization of the particular *chakra* level of consciousness. Each *chakra* sensitizes the person relative to the need inherent in the *chakra*. The first, the base *chakra* (*muladhara*), concerns basic security, safety, and nurturance. The second (*swadhisthana*) has to do with pleasure, sensuality, and sexuality. And the third (*manipura*) involves power and control. These "lower" *chakras* are transcended through the fourth or heart *chakra* (*anahata*), which concerns love. The heart *chakra* is the pivot between the three lower *chakras* and the three higher spiritual *chakras*.

The ethical decision concerning touch should be "No" whenever the touch is a manifestation of a lower-*chakra* need on the part of the therapist. Whenever the therapist is urged to touch by his or her need for security, for erotic stimulation or fulfillment, or for the feeling of personal power and control over the client, that touch should be eschewed. To touch for such reasons, knowingly, is unethical. Furthermore, it is important for the ethical therapist to look deeply and honestly into himself or herself in order to recognize and rectify any inclinations to project these lower-*chakra* needs onto the client (e.g., in the case of projected first-*chakra* needs, to respond with nurturing or reassuring touch). Such touch would, of course, not be in response to the client's needs, but would be a convoluted attempt on the part of the therapist to meet his or her own need. At times, supervision or further therapy may be called for, so that the therapist can recognize and bring under control any tendencies to project personal needs onto clients.

The decision model I am presenting in this chapter takes into consideration both a theoretical dimension and an ethical dimension per se. Touch in psychotherapy is ethical when the theoretical and ethical considerations have *both* been met. In other words, touch in psychotherapy is ethical when the decision to touch is "Yes" on both the theoretical dimension and the ethical dimension.

INFORMED CONSENT FOR TOUCHING

As clarifying and helpful as the ethical decision model may be, I believe that discussion of some additional matters will further elucidate our topic. One such matter is "informed consent." With respect to touching in psychotherapy, "informed consent" means (1) to tell the client of the intention to touch, giving sufficient description of the touch intended and explanation of the rationale for it that the client is truly informed; and (2) to ask, in a noncoercive manner, whether the client consents. Particularly in the early part of therapy, it is advisable to be explicit in seeking informed consent. Also, this is advisable even later on in therapy if the therapist wants to introduce a form of touch that has not been a previous element in the work with this client. As the therapeutic relationship grows, and the therapist and client develop a history of working together, it may become less and less important to seek informed consent. The informed consent may become implicit. The exception to such implicit consent is, as suggested above, the introduction of a new form of touch.

What I have said about informed consent applies primarily to touch as a technique and to touch as expression of the therapeutic relationship. It can, however, be important with socially stereotyped touch or perhaps even with touches as conversational markers. Before hugging a client for the first time, one might do well to ask, "Would you like a good-bye hug?" Or before using conversational markers for the first time, one might say, "I tend to touch sometimes when I am talking personally, as we are doing now. Would that be all right with you?" Of course, any time the client shows the slightest indication of discomfort with a touch, it is wise for the therapist to discuss this with the client in a manner that is in keeping with the relationship of the therapy.

The following are several examples of how I handle informed consent in my work with technical touch and touch as expression of the therapeutic relationship. These are typical of things I say. With a fairly new client who wants to access emotion but is having difficulty, I may say:

> I have an idea of something that may be helpful. I have used this technique a lot with clients, and usually when we do it they access their blocked or inhibited feelings. What I have in mind is for you to lie on your back. I will sit beside you and simply place my hand on your abdomen at about waist level. I will increase the pressure, gradually, over several minutes. Your job is just to lie there and let whatever wants to happen, happen. We may or may not say anything for a few minutes. Would you like to try this?

Or, with a fairly new client who is sobbing, I may say, but only if I genuinely feel it:

> I feel the urge to sit beside you with my arm around you. Would you like that?

In my training workshops, where I am teaching professionals in the use of body-oriented techniques, I use a general statement of informed consent. I say something to this effect before entering into any experiential teaching:

> One of my ground rules in my workshops with professionals is for you each to be your own chairperson. This means, in good Gestalt fashion, to be responsible for yourself. Anything that I suggest for you to do, whether it's a group exercise or something I suggest in a one-on-one demonstration with one of you, is intended as an invitation. As with any genuine invitation, you have the right of refusal. You have the right to enter into the activity to whatever depth feels right to you. If it doesn't feel right to you, just say "No." I will respect any clear "No" that I hear.

With clients who have a history of working with me, and with whom I have a good therapeutic alliance, I abbreviate what would otherwise be intrusive verbiage. With them, informed consent may be only a sentence or two:

> Would you like to try an experiment?

or

> I've got an idea. Would you like to try something?

And with some clients who have a long history of work with me, and with whom I have an unusually good working alliance, I may introduce a technique or may move to touch without a word. The informed consent has become established, implicit in our very work.

Informed consent is important, at core, because it is in keeping with an attitude of respect for the client. The consideration of the therapeutic needs of the client is also a manifestation of this attitude of respect. As I view it, the consideration of the good of the client is the basis of the ethics of psychotherapy. It follows, then, that this is the basis as well for any exposition on the ethics of touch in psychotherapy. And the good of the client is best served through an attitude of profound respect. When the client is regarded with profound respect, ethics will surely be served.

CONCLUDING REFLECTIONS:
ETHICS, LEGALITY, GOOD TASTE, AND GRACE

My attempt here has been to provide a practical guide to the ethics of touch in psychotherapy. I have not explicitly addressed those ethical issues that are the focus of modern philosophy. These issues involve questions of ethical subjectivity or objectivity, questions of whether ethical judgments are true or false or merely the expressions of the feelings of those who utter them and evocative of the feelings of those who hear them (emotivism). They further involve questions of whether an act is to be judged as ethical or unethical on the basis of the motive for the act (motivist theories), the consequence of the act (consequence theories), or the performance of the act out of duty or obligation (deontological theories). I will leave such deep philosophical discussion to those more qualified than I.

However, I do want to distinguish among what is ethical, legal, graceful, and in good taste. Although there is considerable overlap among these categories, what is legal and what is ethical are not identical. A few acts pertaining to the practice of psychotherapy may be proscribed by municipal ordinance or by county, state, or federal law, but may not be in violation of any ethical code. Conversely, most of what is contained in the ethical codes of the helping professions is not covered by law. Therefore, it is possible to be ethical while violating the law, as well as to be legal in one's conduct while in violation of ethical principles. For example, it is not illegal to administer an orgonomic touch to the masseter muscles in order to release the expression of held-back anger. Under some circumstances, however, it may not be ethical, as we have seen. This would be the case if an inadequately trained therapist were to employ the technique, or if the technique were to be used to make the therapist feel powerful. In the case of sexual touch, I have noted earlier that several states have recently enacted laws making it illegal as well as unethical, thereby creating legal–ethical overlap.

Good taste is highly subjective. Beyond the law and beyond the ethical code, good taste pertains to making choices that are not seen by one's peers as lacking in appropriate dignity and professionalism. One area where I see the application of the criterion of good taste as particularly important is in advertising. In compliance with a judgment of the federal government that the American Psychological Association was in violation of fair trade by virtue of its ethical constraints on advertising, the ethical code (American Psychological Association, 1992) now allows advertising. The code now, in essence, requires only that a psychologist not make false statements in advertising. Much room has thus been cleared for tacky behavior. For example, it would be neither illegal nor unethical to erect a large, flashing neon sign announcing one's professional services, as long as no false claims are made. Most members of the profession, however, would surely see this as in poor taste.

Closely related to good taste is gracefulness, but it is even more subjective. "Grace," as I use it here, pertains to a person's conduct in the role of professional. Well beyond the law and the ethical code, and even beyond the judgment of good taste, it involves the skilled use of timing and intensity. Laura Perls once stated that "magic" in psychotherapy is a matter of timing. Speaking too soon or too late reduces the impact of presence. Likewise, intervening with too little or too much intensity misses the mark. The too little or too much, the too soon or too late, constitute awkwardness. The right intensity at just the right time—that is grace.

In teaching about the ethics of psychotherapy, some have suggested what they have termed the "well-lit room principle." The idea is to reflect on one's behavior and intended behavior as if it were happening or about to happen in a well-lit room with one's professional peers observing. What would they say about the behavior? The guideline is to proceed only with the approbation of one's consultants in fantasy.

Our ethics evolve. Societal consciousness changes; the position of psychotherapists in society changes; and research informs us of false beliefs that have been translated into ethical pronouncements. Survey data have suggested that many psychotherapists are more guided in their practice by theory than by empirical findings. As research expands and increases in sophistication, psychotherapy theories may require revision, and this has ethical implication.

In light of the evolving nature of ethics, it is important to consider ethical decisions in the context of the time frame. Some practices that were common a quarter of a century ago (or less) were not then unethical, but now would be. So it is inappropriate to make ethical judgments of practice at one time, based on the standards of another time. The enlightened view is to hold one accountable to the standard of practice that is or was in effect at the time. To do otherwise would violate the *ex post facto* principle of law, which protects one from prosecution for acts performed prior to the time that such acts became legally prohibited.

My purpose in this chapter has been to explore issues relevant to the topic of the ethics of touch in psychotherapy, and to offer a model for making ethical decisions concerning touch. This is no mere casuistry: I am advocating an aspirational ethic based on dispassionate reasoning informed by the facts as we know them. The call is to aspire to touch that is legal, ethical, graceful, and in good taste. In a word, the call is to aspire to impeccability.

REFERENCES

Alyn, J. (1988). The politics of touch in therapy: A response to Willison and Masson. *Journal of Counseling and Development, 66,* 432–433.
American Psychological Association. (1992). Ethical principles of psychologists and code of conduct. *American Psychologist, 47*(4), 1597–1611.
Goodman, M., & Teicher, A. (1988). To touch or not to touch. *Psychotherapy, 25,* 492–500.
Hall, E. T. (1973). *The silent language.* Garden City, NY: Doubleday.
Kupfermann, K., & Smaldino, C. (1987). The vitalizing and revitalizing of experience of reliability: The place of touch in psychotherapy. *Clinical Social Work Journal, 15*(3), 223–235.
Smith, E. (1985). *The body in psychotherapy.* Jefferson, NC: McFarland.
Smith, E. (1992). The ego-syntonic imperative. *Voices, 28*(2), 9–10.
Smith, E. (1994). Anahata, freeze-dried. In E. Tick (Ed), with J. Flossdorf, *My father was Shiva.* Norwood, NJ: Ablex.
Travers, J. (Ed.). (1994). *Psychotherapy and the dangerous patient.* New York: Haworth.
Travers, J. (1995). A harsh and dreadful profession. *Voices, 31*(2), 62–72.
Westbrook, A., & Ratti, O. (1970). *Aikido and the dynamic sphere.* Tokyo: Charles E. Tuttle.

4

A RATIONALE FOR PHYSICAL TOUCHING IN PSYCHOTHERAPY

Reuven Bar-Levav

Our patients in the 1990s are not really sicker than those of the 1890s. But the pace of our life is faster. Our moral and behavioral codes are looser. Our families sustain the individual less well. And we have much more freedom to act out. Vienna of 100 years ago was tight-lipped and straight-laced. The emotional illnesses today are more blatant. We are not treating nice neurotic patients.

It is much clearer now that the basic source of their anxiety is not Oedipal trauma, but the preverbal experiences they had as newborns and infants. For almost 2 years, each of us lived in such darkness before consciousness or memory existed. We had many frightening physical experiences during that time, but no ability to understand any of them. Most of these were objectively safe, but we could not know that. The nerve fibers of our cortex were not yet fully myelinated, and this part of our brain was not yet functional (Bar-Levav, 1988).

But nothing is lost in the universe. We survived, and within us survived traces of those early experiences. For the rest of our days, each of us lives with the same chance physiological response patterns that were associated with our survival. In adulthood we often react as if we were in danger, when in fact no danger exists. Similarly, old hurt and preverbal rage are easily stimulated in adulthood by mildly hurtful or annoying experiences. Our body reacts in the present to signals from another age, long ago. The messages are wrong, but our body does not know it. Such "incorrect" responses are the cause of most adult difficulties and failures. These wrong messages are not sent by the cortex, the organ of understanding. They are issued instead by the subcortical brain, the one that controlled the autonomic nervous system at the very beginning and that sustains life thereafter.

Explanations to the cortex are therefore useless. It is not the source of the trouble and not in charge here. Patients understand, gain insight, and agree with our interpretations and reconstructions, but they do not change as a result. Even in "talking" therapies, the body and its physiological patterns must be altered. Not our thinking.

Until recently this appeared to be an impossible task. How can we ever know what happened before the patient had any memory and any consciousness? We cannot know it from what the patient says. But we can deduce it from what the patient is, and what he or she shows characterologically and characteristically. Our new knowledge of early infant development is also useful.

The basic human experience is universally the same. Individual differences exist only in the details. We know, for instance, why Spitz's babies died in England, even though they never told us. They were not mothered properly. They were carefully attended to, fed, and changed, but this was not enough. And how were they not mothered properly? They were not held and touched enough, and not well enough (Spitz, 1957). They literally wilted and died.

Everything that newborns and infants know about the universe they learn through their physical sensations. Orality is only one route. And not always the most important one. Our sense of safety comes from the softness, firmness, consistency, and steadiness of the mothering body. Most commonly this refers to the biological mother, but not necessarily.

If Mother is immature and anxious, the baby knows its world as jerky and jumpy, or as stifling and crushing. Such mothers typically hold their babies either too loosely lest they be crushed, or too tightly lest they slip and fall. Or Mother might cling to her baby to lessen her own anxiety. Either way, the young organism "knows" the world through such experiences. And this remains its "knowledge" for life, unless it is modified by good, long-term psychotherapy that addresses and changes such physiological expectations.

But how do we address and change such preverbal "knowledge"? Surely not by talking from our cortex to the patient's. It is done by repeatedly establishing exquisite contact with the distrustful and scared infant within the adult patient. We persist until the fragile inner baby begins to feel safe in the therapeutic setting. Only then do patients drop their socially acceptable ways of being and of behaving. The affects and physical reactions of early preverbal experiences then bubble up and come to the surface.

This also happens in marriages, and this is what often destroys them. The expectations that result from the feelings that bubble up are not satisfiable in any reality. And such affects come up in real relationships with compassionate, consistent, and competent psychotherapists who earn the patients' trust over time. But only if a strict non-acting-out contract is in place. Such primitive and powerful affects remain in hiding unless the environment is experienced as totally safe. The emerging affects represent emotional experiences from the period of normal autism soon after birth, and, strictly speaking, they are therefore not transference.

Experiencing such affects early in life or many years later is obviously not the same: Only the adult patient is in a position to observe the panic, the deep hurt, and the extreme rage even while they are bubbling up. This is the critical difference. It makes resolution of the earliest autistic horrors possible. Sooner or later it becomes clear even to very disturbed patients that their enormously powerful storms of affect are not a function of the therapist or of the therapeutic setting. Here it's safe. All is well in reality.

Although propelled by powerful wishes to escape, to withdraw, or to lash out, none of these in fact occur as long as the non-acting-out contract holds. In the meantime the body's musculature, physiology, and subcortical brain are slowly "trained" to recognize that the information imbedded in them is wrong. Not having the powers of observation of the cortex, they are slow learners.

Patients must repeat such affective hurricanes many times before the wrong messages are no longer sent and received. The feelings finally change too. This is the essence of psychotherapy that heals depression. No wonder that such a process is tedious and takes a very long time. But real personality and character change is now an achievable goal. Living essentially without anxiety and depression is possible.

Physical touch, with the explicit permission of the patient each time anew, is the most reassuring intervention when the body undergoes such hurricanes. They are often experienced as literally life-threatening. Every patient naturally always wants to avoid them, or to escape from them as soon as possible. Verbal reassurance is not always enough.

A firm but gentle touch at the right moment allows a patient to endure such experiences of extreme panic and pain without bolting. It intensifies the deep sobbing of hurt. It allows patients not to limit their powerful expressions of rage. These are always very frightening, and especially so for patients who have never had room to express any protest openly. Many people, including professionals, confuse the verbal expression of rage with acts of violence or aggression. They fear losing control. Patients sometimes need a hand, literally, not to curb such safe expressions of rage. Repressing affects cripples effectiveness in general.

The laying on of hands was always considered to be helpful in medicine. It is not hocus-pocus. It is not magic. The scared infant within the sick adult patient was always reassured by the touching hands of a physician. This often saved lives when no specific treatments existed.

Forbidding touch on the basis of the possibility of stimulating an erotic transference essentially reflects the fears in the therapist. Though it is often expressed as a generally accepted fact, such an assumption is also theoretically incorrect. The yearning of a patient for the therapist's love is not sexual. Such yearnings for affection are not even embarrassing when seen for what they really are: yearnings of the panicky infant to be mothered safely and perfectly.

We must make room for such yearnings and welcome their open and full expression. They are a necessary step on the road to self-mothering. Proceeding on this road often requires a gentle, obviously nonsexual, touch on the forearm or on the shoulder. More than any number of wise words, it speaks louder, more clearly, and more directly to the patient's confusion and fear.

ACKNOWLEDGMENT

This chapter is reprinted by permission from the *International Journal of Psychotherapy and Critical Thought,* Vol. 1, No. 1, Fall 1993, pp. 5–7.

REFERENCES

Bar-Levav, R. (1988). *Thinking in the shadow of feelings: A new understanding of the hidden forces that shape individuals and societies.* New York: Simon & Schuster.
Spitz, R. A. (1957). *A genetic field theory of ego formation.* New York: International Universities Press.

RESEARCH PERSPECTIVES

5

RESEARCH ON COMMUNICATION BY TOUCH

Joen Fagan
Alma Smith Silverthorn

When I (Joen Fagan) was in graduate school in the 1950s, there were two ways of doing therapy—psychoanalysis and Rogerian nondirective therapy. (It wasn't even a choice for psychologists, since we were seldom accepted for analytic training.) Little changed until the second half of the 1960s, when a number of powerful new approaches to therapy generated tremendous excitement. As part of this development, together with the general cultural support for experimentation in relationships, touch therapy moved from being taboo to being discussed and used. However, not only was there no research on the effects of touch in therapy; there wasn't even any research on touch communication. This chapter, summarizes an extensive program in which, individually and collectively, I and then-graduate students Alma Smith Silverthorn, Robert Timms, Mildred Allen Broughton, and Patricia Emerson tackled two very difficult-to-research areas: touch and emotion. We devised a procedure that could measure people's ability to understand emotional communications, validated it in standard ways, and then used it to explore a number of interesting hypotheses. The aim of this chapter is to bring the reader along with us in following our thought processes and in sharing the delight of discovery that goes with research, especially in a difficult area that requires innovation.

Most of the specific procedural or statistical details are not included; persons interested in those can ask their libraries to arrange an interlibrary loan of the dissertations on which this chapter is based (see the Acknowledgments and References). Although the research was completed in the early 1970s, there is no reason to believe that it is any less valid today. Indeed, it is doubtful that this research could be conducted at all in today's environment of difficulty in getting approval for "out-of-line" research.

MEASURING WHAT TOUCH MEANS: BEGINNINGS

Our wish to measure how well people understand the "meanings" of touch began as Alma Smith Silverthorn and I talked about the many purposes that could be served if we could measure the accuracy with which people perceive touch. Touch, together with other forms of nonverbal expression (gestures, facial expressions, etc.), is a language, a means of communication. However, we usually think of communication as verbal. There are numerous test instruments to measure verbal skills, and the resulting amount of research is extensive. Vocabulary has been found to be the best measure of IQ, and the accuracy with which people comprehend verbal language is very predictive of success in school and the like. Measuring the language of touch has lagged far behind, for many good reasons. If we could come up with a good "touch IQ" test, what could it predict? We mused that there is much evidence demonstrating that when animal and human babies are deprived of touch in infancy, they do not develop normally, either physically or emotionally. We noted that when people touch, the distance between them decreases, both literally and figuratively. In contrast to seeing and hearing, both of which are distancing and objectifying senses, our world shrinks when we touch. I become much more aware of you and you-and-I and the possibility of emotional involvement. And often touch is what facilitates my joy, sadness, or longing so that deeply held feelings rise to the surface. So, if we could accurately measure how well people understand what is being "said" when they are touched by another—in other words, if we could create a good touch vocabulary test—then we might know much more about the ability to form relationships, and possibly be able to assess the amount of emotional difficulties. Skill with verbal language tells us about "intelligence" as the term is usually understood; we wondered whether skill with touch language would tell us about "relational intelligence" or "emotional intelligence." To be able to answer such questions, we had to devise an instrument that would be stable over time and across persons, and would result in responses that could be objectively scored.

DEVELOPING AN INSTRUMENT

The problem was *how* to measure such idiosyncratic and subtle processes as touch and emotion. We would have to touch people in a nonthreatening way that would not allow information from other senses to be brought to bear. This could be done by asking subjects to put their hands beneath a black curtain on a table, so that they could not see either the person touching their hands or the gestures themselves. We thought of several types of emotional messages that could be communicated by touch and wrote up "scripts" for these, so that our examiners could think about and "feel their way into" the messages they were trying to communicate. For each script, we carefully described appropriate hand movements for the experimenters to make. Finally, to help the subjects tell us what they thought each message was, we created a list of adjectives so that after each message, the subject could mark the adjectives that best described the message. These could be scored based on their accuracy.

We were then ready to try these procedures with live subjects, but with considerable trepidation, since many things could go wrong. We had three questions: Would the subjects accept the procedure? Would they be accurate in selecting adjectives? And would there be a difference in scores among groups that should differ markedly in emotional adjustment? We tested four groups with five subjects in each: nursing students; depressive patients; alcoholic patients (I) who had been hospitalized less than 1 week; and alcoholic patients (II) who had been hospitalized from 3 weeks to 3 months. (We noted that the patients were older, were all males, and had less education than the nurses, but the effects of sex, age, and education could be checked later.) We used three hand messages—one positive/friendly, one neutral, and one negative/angry—each with a script to be read silently by the examiner and "felt into" before the examiner touched the subjects' hands with the specified movements. As noted above, we had devised a list of adjectives that the subjects could choose from to describe each message. And we proceeded. First, the subjects did accept the procedure; no one refused to put his or her hands under a cloth for a faceless stranger to touch. They also marked the adjectives on the list with thought and reasonable accuracy. But these just showed that the procedure was workable. The real excitement came when we looked for differences among the groups and found that the results came out as predicted: Of the adjectives that accurately identified the messages sent by the examiner, the nurses chose 72%, the alcoholics (I) chose 52%, the depressives chose 41%, and the alcoholics (II) chose 32%. We were very encouraged, since the procedure seemed to work and the results were significant in the direction we had predicted.

Now we developed more refined tools. We wrote eight scripts communicating more specific emotions. To develop a more carefully chosen adjective list, we gave the scripts and a list of adjectives to 40 undergraduates (the ubiquitous, Psych 201 students) and asked them to mark the adjectives most descriptive of each message. We included the most frequently chosen five words for each message in the final list.

A testing procedure that can be used by only one person is worthless. So for the next study we used two examiners to see whether they were able to communicate the same message. For subjects, we were fortunate in having available to us graduate psychotherapy students who had had a course in sensory awareness and nonverbal communication. In this course, as part of their therapy training, they had been taught about communicating sympathetic presence through touch, and had experienced inappropriate types of touching (such as intrusive, seductive, and controlling). Attentiveness to their own and others' emotional messages was also emphasized.

Alma tested 20 of these subjects, and another examiner who had been carefully trained in the hand movements tested 8. Since half the subjects were female and half were male, we could now find out whether the gender of the subjects made any difference. Again, the results were encouraging. The correlations between the adjectives chosen by the male and female subjects were high, as were the correlations between the words chosen by the subjects of the two examiners. Because of the training the graduate students had had, we could assume that their responses were probably the most accurate we could get, so we used their responses as the criteria for "correctness" and for our final refinements to the instrument. We weeded out the messages that had produced the lowest correlations and chose the best five for the final instrument: Mothering, Playful, Detached, Fearful, and Angry. (Mothering touch, for example, involved gentle stroking and patting of the back of the hand; Angry touch was expressed by several sudden light but sharp slaps.) We devised a scoring system so that marking five adjectives for each message would result in a maximum score of 10, for a total possible score of 50. Now the instrument was far enough along that we could name it—the Touch Communication Index, or TCI for short.

This was a different kind of test, since it did not employ a paper-and-pencil format; rather, the gestures themselves were the test. It was therefore important to train examiners carefully so that they would do the touches in the same way, and to demonstrate from the subjects' responses that they had been given the same messages. The next study was designed to test this. In addition, we had a number of other questions to answer. So far, we had used only female examiners. Would a male examiner give comparable results? Would there be an examiner–subject gender interaction effect? (I.e., would the various combinations of FF, MM, FM, and MF give similar results?) What about other variables, such as age and marital status? Other things being equal, subjects who were older and married should have accumulated more experience with touching, and if experience per se did make a difference, they should obtain higher scores.

Finally, we found a paper-and-pencil scale that might have some relevance to our efforts. Sidney Jourard, who had done a variety of studies about the things people tell other people, had devised the Body Accessibility Scale, which asked subjects about the parts of their bodies that had been seen or touched in the preceding year by four people: mother, father, male friend, and female friend. Would high scores on this scale be related to high scores on the TCI? To begin answering these questions, we went back to our Psych 201 students, using a female and a male examiner (each of whom tested 10 male and 10 female subjects). We also asked the subjects to complete the Jourard Body Accessibility Scale.

INITIAL RESULTS WITH THE TCI

When we had completed the experiment, checked the scores, and analyzed them statistically, we found several surprises. Age had no significant effect; neither did marital status. The scores on the Body Accessibility Scale showed no relationship at all with the TCI. Encouragingly, there was almost no difference on scores among the four different examiner–subject gender combinations. We also ran correlations between the adjectives checked by the subjects of the two new examiners and the subjects of the original examiner in the first study, and the correlations were high. We were encouraged by the evidence that additional examiners of either sex could be trained to administer the TCI, but we were perplexed that neither our rough measures of cumulative experience nor the Jourard estimate of frequency of touching and being touched showed significant effects. However, we went back to our parallel with verbal intelligence and noted that, within broad limits, age in adulthood and marital status have little effect on IQ.

Continuing to be both encouraged and intrigued, we set up another study. This time we asked in a more rigorous way whether emotional problems had an effect on the TCI. We obtained subjects who were inpatients in a psychiatric hospital: 20 diagnosed as alcoholic, 20 as depressed, and 20 as schizophrenic. We tabulated the length and number of previous hospitalizations, and noted whether the patients were on tranquilizing drugs. The Psych 201 subjects from the previous study served as our control group. In addition to the main question, we could recheck age and marital status, and see whether education level (which should be related to both intelligence and socioeconomic status) had an effect.

Once again, the results were edifying. The college students, with a mean score of 29.6 (out of 50), were significantly more accurate than the three psychiatric groups, whose scores ranged from 20.4 to 22.7. All four groups were most accurate in recognizing the Angry, Playful, and Mothering messages, and least accurate in recognizing Detached. (Detached showed the biggest discrepancy in meaning between groups; the adjectives chosen most frequently by the college students were "indifferent" and "detached," whereas the patients chose "calm" and "peaceful.") In general, the psychiatric group showed a general lowering of accuracy, with more variability in the adjectives chosen. Interestingly, inspection of the responses showed that the errors were not random, but that the psychiatric groups chose adjectives that skewed toward less threatening, less intense emotional meaning. Mothering slid toward "friendly," Angry toward "excited," and Detached toward "calm." Of the other variables, none was significant. Whether the patients were on psychotropic medication made no difference; neither did age, education level, marital status, or length of hospitalization.

There was one more question we wanted to explore at this point. So far, emotional disturbance was the only characteristic that had had an effect on scores. If age, education, and general experience had no effect, would it be possible that specific training in emotional communication might? We set up one final study, going back to our Psych 201 subject pool. Two groups of 11 subjects were used. One group was simply retested after a 1-month interval; the second group participated in weekly sensitivity group training, involving small-group discussion about feelings and verbal expression of feeling responses toward other participants. No specific training involving physical contact was given. On the retest, the control group showed a gain of 3 points, while the experimental group showed an increase of 7—a significant difference. The test—retest correlations were .45 and .53 for the two groups, somewhat lower than would be considered desirable.

As we looked over what we had learned so far, it seemed clear that the TCI had both face and predictive validity, and that different experimenters could be trained to give comparable results. The main problem seemed to be the low reliability, as shown in the final experiment. It was true that we had been randomly varying the order of presentation of the messages, and it was possible that starting with the more subtle messages (Mothering and Detached) might have made it harder to "catch on," especially if the subjects were anxious. (Clammy hands were not infrequent, although no subject ever had refused to finish the testing.) For that reason, we decided on a standard order of presentation—Playful, Angry, Fearful, Mothering, and Detached.

Overall, we were very pleased. The procedures we had devised had overcome several of the problems that had marred most other studies of emotion, such as the discrepancy between real-life emotions (which are hard to arrange and measure) and emotions generated by limited or artificial material. Our adjective list made it easy for subjects to answer and give a range of responses to a specific emotional communication, in a way that could be easily scored.

DEVELOPMENT OF ADDITIONAL TESTS

At this point, Alma left with a well-earned PhD in hand, while I continued. I devised three other tests of emotional communication. First, I filmed the TCI so that I could compare visual cues with the tactile ones. Using the film with the adjective list, I found that our psychology graduate students who had taken the course in sensory awareness performed about equally well on the TCI and the film of it. However, the Psych 201 students scored higher on the film, showing a relative deficit in recognizing tactile cues. (Thanks to TV, college students now have had thousands of hours of recognizing filmed emotional communication, however poor their education in touch may be.)

A second test was based on the work of Davitz (1964), who studied communication by metaphor. Using the same five emotional messages as those in the TCI, I chose several metaphoric statements for each one. For example, for Playful, one of the descriptions was "Bubbles of champagne." Again, subjects were asked to mark five adjectives from the list.

A third test was also based on Davitz's (1969) work, this one using statements about body feelings for each of the five emotions. An example of a body statement for Playful was "I feel wide awake."

The group of graduate students with the sensory awareness training also scored higher on the Metaphor Scale and the Body Scale than the Psych 201 subjects. The correlations between the four instruments were generally low, suggesting that skill in "reading" the emotions communicated by touch, visual cues, metaphoric statements, and body feelings may require different skills, learnings, or personality characteristics.

PERSONALITY CHARACTERISTICS
OF HIGH AND LOW SCORERS

Bob Timms now began a series of studies to explore the difference in personality factors between good and poor receivers of emotional communication. In addition to the TCI, Bob used the three other measures of emotional communication that I had devised: the Metaphor Scale, the Body Scale, and the Film of Touch, together with two widely used personality measures: the Minnesota Multiphasic Personality Inventory (MMPI) and the Rokeach Value Survey. Four groups of subjects were available, ranging from minimal to severe in the degree of their emotional difficulty. The four groups were medical patients undergoing physical rehabilitation, psychosomatic patients, neurotic anxiety patients, and alcoholics. There were 20 subjects in each group, for a total of 80; all were hospitalized, the age range was from 20 to 50, and the education range was from 7 to 12 years.

On all four of the communication tests, the physical rehabilitation and psychosomatic groups scored significantly higher than the neurotic and alcoholic groups. Most of the correlations between the four tests were positive and significant, ranging from .36 to .68. In general, the correlations between the Metaphor Scale and the other tests were lower, suggesting a degree of relationship between the more body-oriented measures that was not fully shared by the more abstract Metaphor Scale.

To explore personality differences between high and low scorers on the four tests, the highest five scorers and the lowest five scorers on each one were chosen from each of the four diagnostic groups. We chose this way so as not to overload or bias the results; otherwise, the low scorers would have come largely from the neurotic and alcoholic groups. Then an analysis was performed on the 13 scales of the MMPI for the high- and low-scoring groups. The TCI, the Body Scale Test, and the Film of Touch had six, eight, and seven significantly different MMPI scales for the respective tests, all of these in a more deviant or pathological direction for the low scorers. The Metaphor Scale had three significantly different MMPI scales. The scales that most frequently distinguished between the high- and low-scoring groups were the *F* scale (which measures deviance of response) and Schizophrenia, with Paranoia, Psychasthenia, Hypomania, and Hypochondriasis next.

We then looked at the individual items on the MMPI. Of the large number that were significantly different, almost all were answered in the deviant direction by the low-scoring group. The items seemed to group into several categories. Low scorers reported themselves as being suspicious of others; withdrawing from social contact; having family problems; having many physical complaints; and feeling guilty, depressed, and anxious. Those with low scores specifically on the TCI reported bizarre experiences, showed very strong withdrawal tendencies, and had sexual difficulties, so it seemed clear why they would have trouble understanding touch messages.

A commonly used scale consisting of a number of items from the MMPI is the Ego Strength scale. On this, we found the most profound difference between our high and low scorers. The high-scoring group endorsed between 23 and 42 items; the low-scoring group endorsed between 0 and 18. In psychological studies, it is rare to get results that show such a clear separation without any overlap. This was an impressive confirmation that receiving the feelings accurately of others was strongly related to ego strength.

On the Rokeach Value, the results were not so clear-cut. When combined, the four low-scoring groups all ranked two of the values— national security and obedience—significantly higher than the high scorers, who ranked pleasure and independence higher. The value pattern here seemed to represent the authoritarian personality type versus a more libertarian approach.

A final part of the study reexamined Alma's earlier finding that scores could improve after sensitivity training. This time Bob retested the 20 physical rehabilitation patients after they had received 6 weeks of intensive physical therapy, which included massage and other procedures involving touch. Although the main purpose of this therapy was to assist the patients in recovery and in regaining bodily functioning, it would certainly seem that this amount of skilled, caring touch should increase openness to touch messages. There was significant improvement on the TCI, and also on the Body and Film Scales, but not on the Metaphor Scale. The physical therapists also were retested after 6 weeks, but showed no significant increase in scores.

In summary, Bob's studies supported the previous findings that persons with fairly severe emotional difficulties were less accurate in receiving emotional communication than persons with only mild or moderate emotional difficulties, no matter which of the four tests was used. Certain personality characteristics, such as the inability to share emotional experiences, inhibition, anxiety, and focus on physical problems, were related to reduced accuracy in receiving and understanding emotional communication. Value orientations were less important, and improvement in accuracy was possible through the physical contact that is a part of physical therapy.

In all the research to this point, the TCI differentiated among severely disturbed, moderately disturbed, normal, and sophisticated subjects. The differences between the high and low scorers were large and convincing.

TESTING OF SCHIZOPHRENICS

Millie Broughton was interested in the then-current theory about emotional communication and schizophrenia—the "double-bind" theory that Haley, Bateson, Mehrabian, and a number of other authors had proposed. Essentially, these authors suggested that schizophrenia is a disorder of communication involving the giving of two contradictory messages at the same time. They had observed that this was a common form of communication in the families of schizophrenics. In such incongruent communication, positive messages such as "I like you" are accompanied by a tone of voice or a facial expression that simultaneously gives a very different message, leaving the recipient no good way to respond even while a response is expected or required. The more elegant way of stating this is that inappropriate affect and incongruent emotional messages result in psychopathology. Such confused and disordered communication over time produces an inability to discriminate reality and to understand the emotional messages of others, as well as one's own feelings. Double-bind theory also hypothesizes that schizophrenics, compared to "normals," are less able to discriminate conflicting emotional messages, are more sensitive to negative emotions, attend more to nonverbal cues than to verbal cues, and are more able to understand metaphor than body messages.

At the time, the evidence for all of these hypotheses had been largely clinical and/or anecdotal. Having the four tests with similar messages on visual and tactile channels (and since I had also made tapes of the messages, we could present them auditorily) made it possible for the first time to give an experimental answer to the double-bind hypotheses. Millie designed her study to ask whether schizophrenic subjects differed from normal subjects in their ability to discriminate the following:

1. Emotions transmitted through three different sensory channels (tactile, visual, and auditory).

2. Emotions transmitted through (a) one channel, (b) two channels carrying consistent messages, or (c) two channels carrying inconsistent messages.
3. Five different emotional messages, varying from positive to negative.

In addition, three paper-and-pencil tests were used. These measured how much people wished to be held (Hollender), whether they maximized or minimized sensory input (the Spiegel Personality Inventory), and whether they responded more to visual or to verbal materials (Shapiro). Millie tested 40 Psych 201 undergraduates (who served as her "normal" group) and 40 diagnosed schizophrenics, 32 who were hospitalized and 8 outpatients. As far as possible, subjects were chosen so as not to be chronic.

There was a significant difference between the normal and schizophrenic groups on all three channels, regardless of whether the communication was consistent or inconsistent. However, the schizophrenic subjects showed no greater problem with inconsistent messages than the normal subjects did; there was no interaction of diagnosis and inconsistent communication. This failure to support the hypotheses was disappointing for us at the time. We were surprised that this study did not support the double-bind hypotheses, and were not satisfied with our explanations of the negative findings. More recently, as our knowledge of brain chemistry has increased, schizophrenia has come to be regarded as a disorder of neurotransmission, with some genetic basis. So, although the results of this study were confusing at the time, the lack of relevance of double-bind communications as a causative factor of schizophrenia has been substantiated by later research.

There were other interesting findings from our research. When the two presented messages were inconsistent, the Fearful message took precedence over any other message and was "heard" most clearly. The Playful and Mothering messages were responded to more accurately than the Detached message. For both groups, there was a difference in which channels carried the most impact: Auditory messages were received most strongly, followed by tactile and then visual. As predicted, the schizophrenic group's average score was slightly higher than the control group's on the Metaphor Scale—the only test where this occurred. On the three pencil-and-paper tests, persons who had an aversion to sensory stimulation tended to be less receptive to emotional communication. Also, as subjects indicated more need for physical contact, their scores on the Body Scale increased.

In summary, schizophrenic subjects were less accurate than control subjects in the reception of emotional communication, whether presented on one sensory channel or two, whether consistent or inconsistent, and whether positive or negative; the exception of was metaphoric communication. When presented with inconsistent communication in different emotional channels, both groups in this study attended more to what they heard than what they saw or felt. Fear took priority over other messages. Finally, receiving emotional communication accurately was negatively related to minimizing sensory input and positively related to acknowledged need for physical contact.

RELIABILITY AND CORRELATIONS WITH OTHER VARIABLES

A final study by Patricia Emerson tackled several unanswered questions. The main one was test–retest reliability; others were the relationship between TCI scores and intelligence, mood states, and personality variables.

Previous test–retest correlations were .45, .53, .58, and .55—low enough to reduce the value of the test. To try to increase reliability to a more acceptable level, Patricia tried a new form of answer sheet. The old adjective list had several problems. It required subjects to scan rapidly down the page, making it easy to overlook items; in addition, only a few items from a large list were used in the scoring. Patricia's new form used a separate page of adjectives for each of the five messages. Thirty pairs were presented, and the subject had to choose the most descriptive adjective in each pair. A pilot study was done to choose specific adjectives. Then 22 subjects were tested at a 1-week interval for a test–retest reliability of .59; 21 of these were retested after 1 month for a reliability of .69. Following this, we did an item analysis to assess internal consistency, and some changes were made in scoring.

Now, to assess reliability, 100 Psych 201 subjects were tested using the new adjective form. (We actually tested a total of 116 subjects to allow for dropouts.) Half were retested after 1 week and half after 1 month. In addition, tests were given to assess intelligence, mood, and emotional stability or adjustment. In all the previous testing, subjects varied not only in degree of psychopathology, but also on intelligence, test sophistication, and a number of other factors. Using only students provided a more homogeneous group. The tests used included the Scholastic Aptitude Test, the Profile of Mood States, an adjective checklist, and the Meyers–Briggs Type Indicator. All had been standardized on college students and/or designed for use with them. Two examiners were used, one female and one male.

Overall, the reliability was better with the new scoring system. The reliability on retesting after 1 week was .71 and after 1 month was .64. There was a small but significant increase in the total scores. In looking at other variables, we found a significant effect from the examiners: The male experimenter proved to be less consistent than the female. Again, this finding emphasizes the need for very good training, since the examiner *is* the test.

The effects of intelligence on the TCI were negligible, and mood also showed little effect. Some patterns were apparent on the scales of adjustment and on personality factors. Low scorers were more oriented toward work and liked to deal with facts, whereas high scorer tended to like to play and were more oriented toward people. There were also low correlations between scores on the five messages and various personality scales. Playful was related to affiliation, adjustment, and nurturance; Angry was linked with aggression, succorance, and exhibitionism; Fearful was related to reduced vigor; Mothering was linked with difficulty with endurance; and Detached was correlated with low vigor, low endurance, low achievement, and low order. On the Meyers–Briggs, Intuitive and Feeling types scored higher than Sensing and Thinking types.

In summary, the reliability of the TCI was considerably improved. With carefully trained examiners, it could be expected that scores would be stable. However, it was not clear whether the new scoring sheet had changed the characteristics of the test to some extent. In contrast to all the other studies, no relationship to the level of adjustment was found. Whether this was because the new answer sheet changed the TCI, because the range of adjustment was much smaller for college students, or because of other factors, we didn't know. In retrospect, we wished we had given the MMPI as one of the tests so that we could see whether it would prove more sensitive, and so that we could use Bob's results for comparison.

CONCLUDING THOUGHTS

Let us now look back at what was accomplished in this research program. We demonstrated that it was possible to design a test that could measure a very difficult area, to give this test adequate reliability and validity, and to use it to get useful information. Our negative results concerning the role of the double-bind theory with schizophrenics is a good example of how science operates: A negative result often provides as much information as a positive one, although we may not understand it as readily and may have to wait for the development of other technologies for validation of our results.

Until the last study, we found on every occasion that degree of psychopathology made a big difference in how accurately our subjects understood touch communication. A long-standing finding in many psychological studies is that psychotic and mental hospital patients give poorer responses than normal subjects, possibly as a function of their preoccupations, cognitive problems, or lack of motivation. Were our results a function of this? A part of the answer can be found by looking for patterns. Our early study suggested a patterned shift in meaning; Millie's subjects, as predicted, scored higher than controls on the Metaphor Scale; Bob's study, analyzing both the MMPI scale patterns and the individual items, found clear indications of meaning. All these findings together suggested that the lower scores of subjects with severe emotional problems were not due to random effects. We also know now from several studies that many patients with severe emotional problems have also experienced physical and/or sexual abuse as children—one more reason for them to misinterpret touch. On the other hand, people who are comfortable with their bodies, with touching, and with being touched have fewer emotional problems and understand others more accurately when they communicate about feelings and relationships. Stated this way, it sounds obvious—but testing and experimentation are ways of testing the obvious to make sure we aren't fooling ourselves. When we have such evidence for the obvious, we are able to provide grounding and support for therapeutic practices. On the basis of this series of studies, we can say that the ability to understand emotional communication from others as communicated by touch is an important component of mental health. From there, it is only a small step to posit that therapists, who assume the responsibility to help people become better adjusted and more emotionally stable, should be able to help their patients' translate touch into understandable messages. Therapists may have more trouble accomplishing their therapeutic tasks if they cannot use touch to help people become more comfortable with and knowledgeable about this most basic area of emotional communication.

ACKNOWLEDGMENTS

This chapter is based on the doctoral dissertations of Alma Smith Silverthorn (1970), Robert J. Timms (1971), and Mildred Allen Broughton (1971), and on the master's thesis and doctoral dissertation of Patricia Emerson (1973, 1974).

REFERENCES

Broughton, M. A. (1971). *Perception of consistent and inconsistent affect in normal and schizophrenic subjects.* Unpublished doctoral dissertation, Georgia State University.

Davitz, J. R. (1964). *The communication of emotional meaning.* New York: McGraw-Hill.

Davitz, J. R. (1969). *The language of emotion.* New York: Academic Press.

Emerson, P. (1973). *Effects of awareness training.* Unpublished master's thesis, Georgia State University.

Emerson, P. (1974). *The Tactile Communication Index: Reliability and validity studies.* Unpublished doctoral dissertation, Georgia State University.

Smith, A. (1970). *Non-verbal communication through touch.* Unpublished doctoral dissertation, Georgia State University.

Timms, R. J. (1971). *The ability to receive emotional communication in medical and psychiatric patients.* Unpublished doctoral dissertation, Georgia State University.

DIFFERENCES BETWEEN THERAPISTS WHO TOUCH AND THOSE WHO DO NOT

Judy Milakovich

In these days, when the whole of psychotherapy is being challenged to prove its worth and to improve its efficiency, it seems even more imperative to investigate openly the potential benefits of using non-erotic touch in the therapeutic process. Those of us who use body- and touch-oriented techniques know of their power to transform difficult and chronic psychological problems and to break through impasses. In addition to the effectiveness of these techniques, a growing portion of the public is becoming insistent on approaches to healing that take into account the whole of their being.

The dilemmas for the individual therapist are these: How does one know whom to touch, when, and in what ways? How and when does touching facilitate the therapeutic process, and when does it not? When and how can touch be detrimental to the client, the therapist, or the process? These questions do not yet have answers outside a particular therapists' own intuition and experience. Thus, the ultimate dilemma is the lack of objective knowledge.

Therapists' own experiential, intuitive knowing usually seems a perfectly adequate basis for decision making about touching. However, the legal system, which presumes to pass judgment on therapists' decision making, does not operate on a basis of experiential, intuitive knowing. One of the ways a therapeutic practice is judged ethical or not is by comparing it against "standards of practice." Touch has been, for the most part, a hidden practice, and standards for its use are not available. Managed care companies and health maintenance organizations demand to see the data. A positive result of third-party interest in how psychotherapists do what they do could be that if the efficacy of touch techniques can be empirically proven, such techniques will be supported.

PREVIOUS RESEARCH

Reviewing the research on nonerotic touching in therapy, I found that most of it took place in the more permissive atmosphere of the 1960s, 1970s, and early 1980s. This research, however, tended to be based on a very limited and misleading view of how and why touching occurs in real, ongoing psychotherapy. The studies I found used one-time interview situations and artificial incidents of touch. All used students or actresses and actors as "clients" and "counselors." None of the studies considered such important factors as the state of the therapeutic alliance, the phase of the therapy, or the intention of the touching (see, e.g., Alagna, Whitcher, Fisher, & Wicas, 1979; Suiter & Goodyear, 1985).

In none of the studies was the intention for the touching derived from a psychotherapeutic theoretical perspective. The "clients" did not request to be touched, nor were they consulted about their concerns or wishes about being touched. The form the touching took (arm, leg, shoulder) was casual and of the type that might occur between people in normal social situations. No rationale for the touching was given to the "client," and no processing of the experience occurred. Also, in none of the research was attention paid to the personal characteristics of the therapist doing the touching. Such factors as the therapist's beliefs (both personal and theoretical) about touching, and the amount of training received in touch-oriented therapeutic rationale and technique, have not been considered. The greatest part of the literature concerning the use of touch in therapy is in the form of case histories and theoretical opinion (Horner, 1973; Kupfermann & Smaldino, 1987).

A notable exception is a study by Pope, Tabachnick, and Keith-Spiegel (1987), which shows that therapists of differing theoretical orientations have very different beliefs about the effects of touching clients. These authors found that 30% of humanistic therapists thought that nonerotic hugging, kissing, and affectionate touching might frequently be of benefit to clients' treatment. Only 6% of psychodynamic therapists thought so. The majority of psychodynamic therapists thought that such behavior would be misunderstood, whereas the majority of humanistic therapists thought it would rarely be misunderstood. A major aim of my own study was to discover how therapists come to hold such different beliefs.

OBJECTIVES, SAMPLE, AND METHODS OF THE STUDY

The two main objectives of my study were (1) to identify factors that may differentiate therapists who touch from those who do not touch their clients in individual psychotherapy, and (2) to describe characteristics of psychotherapy practices where nonerotic touch is used as part of the therapeutic process. The first objective was intended to make an initial inquiry into what sorts of events or experiences influence a therapist's decision to touch or not to touch clients. The second objective was intended to give a clearer picture of what factors might be relevant when research into the effects of touch in psychotherapy is considered. The remainder of this chapter reports on the findings from the investigation of the first objective.

The specifics of my study were as follows. A cross-sectional sample of 84 therapists was interviewed for the study. The interviews were done by phone, using a structured questionnaire that had been sent to each therapist prior to the interview. The questionnaire contained 112 questions; 8 of these were open-ended.

The sample was obtained by starting with two sources of participants and then using the snowball method to generate more participants. Equal numbers of male and female therapists were solicited from two sources: (1) The Fielding Institute's electronic network, and (2) my professional associates. Each therapist completing the interview was asked to supply names of colleagues who might be willing to be interviewed. None of the therapists who completed the interview were known personally by me.

The sample included approximately equal numbers of humanistic and psychoanalytic therapists, plus a number of therapists with cognitive and "other" orientations. The average age was 45, and the average amount of experience was 13 years. There were no significant differences across gender for any of the demographic variables or for the variables related to therapeutic practice (years of experience, practice setting, theoretical orientation, degree, number of clients seen, or amount of personal therapy). The only significant difference related to therapist gender was that male therapists saw significantly more male clients than did female therapists. These results made it possible to assume that the gender differences found on the other variables tested were not confounded by demographic and practice characteristics of the sample.

Since my sample was not random, I compared sample characteristics (age, years of experience, amount of personal therapy, theoretical orientation, percentage in private practice) with those in two studies (Pope et al., 1987; Prochaska & Norcross, 1983) that each randomly sampled over 400 American Psychological Association Division 29 members. There were no significant differences between the current sample and the two comparison samples on any of the characteristics, except that my sample had a much higher percentage of humanistically oriented therapists. Perhaps both my sampling technique and the study requirement that two-thirds of the sample touch their clients explain this difference.

An interesting "problem" occurred, as it proved very difficult to find therapists who did not touch their clients at all. Only one of the therapists never touched his clients in any way. This and other results from my study suggest that those of us who touch clients may not be as much in the minority as we may think. Because of this "problem," when I tested the hypotheses, those therapists who touched clients *only* at times of greeting, parting, or termination were defined as therapists who did not touch clients. It could be argued that this is a "weak" definition of therapists who do not touch clients. This is undoubtedly true. It is also possible that such a weak definition makes the differences found between therapist groups even more significant.

PROFESSIONAL AND PERSONAL EXPERIENCES WITH TOUCH IN THERAPY

The results of my study showed that both professional and personal experiences with touch in therapy appeared to influence a therapist's beliefs about touching clients. I hypothesized that having "permission to touch" might be a factor that influenced a therapist's choice about touching clients. I assumed that such permission might come from several sources. In regard to professional experiences, I asked therapists if they had had teachers and/or supervisors who advocated touch as a legitimate practice. I also asked how much training they had in therapeutic modalities that use touch. In regard to personal experiences, I asked if they had personally tried, in either therapy or workshops, different types (I listed seven types and "others") of body-oriented psychotherapy, such as psychomotor and neo-Reichian therapy. And I asked about experiences with being touched by their own therapists.

Professional Experiences

If therapists had received permission to touch clients from either teachers or supervisors, they were significantly ($p < .0001$) more likely to touch their own clients. Sixty percent of the therapists had had a supervisor or teacher who valued touching clients as a legitimate therapeutic practice. Of those who indicated that they had such permission, 70.4% did touch their clients.

The obvious explanation for these results is that the therapists who touch clients have received *explicit* permission to touch from those in positions of authority. Giving permission also conveys implicit beliefs and values about the use of touch in therapy. Teachers/supervisors teach their opinions about theory and about which therapeutic techniques they consider beneficial. In so doing, they convey their underlying beliefs and values about what is needed to ameliorate psychopathology and what is not, and what is therapeutic and what is not.

The choice about touching clients was also significantly ($p < .0001$) associated with having had training in modalities that use touch. Significantly more therapists who didn't touch clients said that they had zero or only a few hours of training in body-oriented psychotherapies. Many therapists who did touch clients reported that they had 50 or more hours of training. It seems obvious that therapists who receive training in modalities that involve touching would feel that they have competence and permission to touch clients. However, it is also possible that therapists who are predisposed toward an interest in touch might be more likely to pursue such training. They might also tend to seek out personal experiences via body therapies, body psychotherapies, and their personal psychotherapy.

Personal Experiences

I asked therapists about how many different types of body therapies, such as massage, Rolfing, or acupuncture, they had tried. The results showed that those therapists who touched their clients were significantly ($p = .005$) more likely to have tried seven or more different body therapies. The number of different experiences therapists had with body-oriented psychotherapies (in workshops or personal therapy) was also significantly ($p = .002$) associated with whether or not they touched clients. Therapists with three or more such experiences were significantly more likely to touch clients than those with fewer than three such experiences.

I also asked therapists about how often they had been touched in their own personal therapy. Eighty-three percent of the female therapists and 55% of the male therapists indicated they had received at least some touch from up to three of their own therapists. Significantly (p = .005) more female therapists than male therapists were touched by their therapists. Eighty-two percent of the therapists reported that they liked the touching they had received from their own therapists, whereas 11% reported that they disliked it; the remaining 7% either did not think the touching they received was significant enough to rate, or felt neutral about their therapists' touch.

Those therapists who liked the touching they had received from their therapists were significantly (p < .0001) more likely to touch clients. Those therapists who were never or only rarely touched by their own therapists touched their clients significantly less often. Interestingly, the amount of touching done by therapists who disliked the touching of their own therapists did not appear to be influenced by their negative experience. Just as many therapists who disliked the touching from their own therapists touched clients as did not touch clients.

Therapists' experiences with personal therapy thus appear to serve as a model for their own therapeutic practices. The experiential understanding of the benefit of a therapeutic practice may serve as a powerful motivation for including the practice in one's own repertoire. The responses to the open-ended questions supported this idea further. Several therapists who had found their own therapists' touch to be beneficial said that they wanted to provide similar experiences for their clients. Some therapists who had not been touched by their therapists said that they did not touch because their therapists had not touched them.

There are certain clinical implications of this explanation. If it is true that therapists want to do for their clients what was done for them, then it is possible that a therapist might misjudge the needs of a particular client. At this point there are no clearly substantiated guidelines about when and when not to use touch, so careful consideration of one's motivation is warranted.

Summary

Professional and personal experiences with touch in therapeutic situations appear to have powerful effects on beliefs and values about the benefit of touch in therapy. The findings reported above suggest that these therapists learned values and beliefs about touching clients from their teachers and supervisors and from their experiences with training and personal therapy. The responses given to open-ended questions about how they thought about touching clients also indicated that therapists who touched clients in nonerotic ways and those who did not had different values and beliefs about the need and benefit of nonerotic touch in therapy. I discuss these next.

DIFFERENCES IN VALUES AND BELIEFS

Answers given to open-ended questions revealed that therapists who touched their clients had beliefs and values about touching clients that differed distinctly from those of therapists who did not touch their clients. Therapists who touched clients said that they thought touching was therapeutically beneficial and sometimes necessary for healing. They also stated that not touching certain clients could be detrimental and unethical. For example, one therapist said, "Touch is therapeutically important. It is the most effective means with some clients. I think it is unethical in these cases to *not* touch the client." Another said, "To refuse to touch in a good way could be detrimental. I deal mostly with abused clients."

These therapists thought that some clients had a "need" for physical nurturing, or a touch "deficit" that was developmental. Many of these therapists mentioned that they thought some clients, especially those who had been sexually abused, needed to experience "safe" touch. They believed that touching such clients could show them that touch could occur within boundaries and that it was not always sexual. One therapist stated, "I have a personal value that people need physical nurturing," and "Touch-deprived (skin hunger) clients need touch." Another said, "I touch to give nurture and support, and to give a physical anchor if they're going through past trauma. I do this especially for those [clients who as children] had adults standing by and watching but not doing anything." And a third said, "Basically, I work with sex abuse clients and I want them to experience safe touching."

These therapists also often mentioned that they personally enjoyed touching and felt comfortable touching clients. Several mentioned that they had been touched by their own therapists and had found it beneficial for them. Many of the therapists who expressed the beliefs outlined above reported that they had been sexually and/or physically abused themselves. (I will return later to the issue of the effects of a personal history of abuse on therapists' decisions about touching.)

Therapists who did not touch their clients had a different set of beliefs and values about touching clients. They believed touching clients to be therapeutically detrimental. They thought that touch was confusing, that it blurred the boundaries between themselves and their clients, and that it was likely to be misperceived. One such therapist said, "I don't touch because of transference aspects, largely. And because of the blurring of boundaries." Another said, "I don't touch because it presents a confusing situation and blurs the boundaries of the therapy."

These therapists also felt that touch was too complex to analyze and that it would encourage dependence. They believed that touch would interfere with treatment goals, in the sense that it took away the client's opportunity to understand his or her own motivations for wanting touch. Thus, they believed that gratifying a client's wish for touch would contaminate the therapy. One therapist said, "Touching interferes with treatment goals. I'm trying to get the client[s] to work independently; I don't want them to depend on me." And another said, "I don't touch because my understanding of the dynamics of acting out feelings versus understanding feelings is that acting out is a good way of not understanding. My job is to help the patient understand. I think touch in therapy is not therapeutic."

These therapists spoke of clients' "wishes" for touch, never calling these "needs." They believed that touching, especially with touch-abused clients, was invasive and would further traumatize them; thus, it would make the therapeutic process unsafe. A few also believed that touching invited the client to sexualize the relationship. These responses are illustrative: "I don't touch because of what it does to patients; I don't want to traumatize them." "I think touch can be invasive. My contract doesn't include touching; it does include the right to be invasive about questions." "Psychoanalysis works when an impulse is frustrated. 'Talk, don't act,' allows an exploration of wishes to find their meaning."

A few of these therapists said that they were personally uncomfortable with touching clients. The therapists with these beliefs also did not mention being touched in their own therapy. None of the therapists with these beliefs reported having been sexually abused. A few did report physical abuse. (The issue of abuse will be discussed in more detail later.)

DIFFERENCES IN PERCEPTIONS OF RISK
AND IN REASONS FOR TOUCH DECISIONS

In an open-ended question, I asked whether therapists thought that touching clients was risky ethically or legally, and what made them willing to touch clients if they did this, or what made them choose not to touch clients. The vast majority of the therapists who touched clients thought that touching was not risky for them. Some said they had never thought about the risks. Many were aware of risks but found these risks acceptable, usually because they trusted themselves to be appropriate. Some said that they simply refused to be controlled by fear.

As noted above, a number of the therapists said that they thought some clients needed touch, and some of them even felt that not touching could be detrimental. Such factors made them willing to touch clients even if they perceived some risks in doing so. One therapist stated, "I touch because some clients need it. I've never had a negative experience. I personally feel grounded and trust myself about doing it well. I don't always trust other professionals." Another therapist said, "I am very aware of possible misunderstandings. I'm very careful, limit my touching, and always ask."

Therapists who did not touch clients gave several reasons for not touching. Most often mentioned was that their theoretical orientation discouraged it. Legal concerns and disapproval by supervisors were mentioned by a few. One such therapist reported, "I'm influenced by the public and professional setting about legal and ethical issues. Touch is easily misinterpreted. The supervisor I use, usually around sexual issues, would be very disturbed if I touched."

Though legal issues were cited by some as the reason for not touching clients, these were not often mentioned and were never mentioned as the only reasons. As in the quote above, other influences (e.g., a conservative community and supervisors' beliefs) were included as reasons for not touching.

As noted earlier, some nontouching therapists thought that touch was invasive, "contaminated" the therapy, and made the therapeutic process unsafe. Others cited the belief that touch was easily misunderstood and produced problems they didn't want to deal with, such as dependence. Still another reason for not touching was personal preference. One therapist said, "I don't feel touch is risky legally or ethically; this is not a concern for me. I don't touch because of my own personality; I only like to be touched by those I know well."

REPORTS OF A PERSONAL HISTORY
(VS. NO HISTORY) OF ABUSE

Although it is understandable that therapists who feel a sense of permission to touch clients and who have learned to value touch as a therapeutic practice do touch clients, it is not enough to explain why some therapists believe touch is particularly beneficial (or even neces-sary) and some do not. My findings show that some therapists who have experienced touch from their own therapists, some who have had teachers and supervisors who advocate touch, and some who have received at least some training in modalities that use touch still choose not to touch clients.

While doing the interviews, I began to observe that a large percentage of the therapists reported sexual and physical abuse expe-riences, and that the majority of these therapists touched their clients. All therapists interviewed were asked a series of questions about possible physical and sexual abuse.

Therapists were first asked whether they thought they had been physically or sexually abused as children and as adults. They indicated the frequency of abuse they felt they had suffered on a 5-point Likert scale from "never" to "often." Forty-five percent of the therapists indicated that they had been physically abused at some time in their lives. However, physical abuse was not statistically associated with whether or not a therapist touched, or did not touch, his or her clients.

Forty-five percent of the therapists indicated that they had been sexually abused at some point in their lives. Although there was no difference in the number of male and female therapists reporting sexual abuse as children, significantly ($p < .0001$) more female therapists than male therapists reported being sexually abused as adults. The data showed that significantly ($p < .0001$) more female therapists who were sexually abused as children were also sexually abused as adults. This finding was not true for male therapists: Sexual abuse as a child and as an adult were linked for females but not for males.

Whether or not a therapist reported a history of sexual abuse, and whether or not a therapist touched his or her clients, were found to be significantly related. What was most interesting was the nature of the associations. *Not* having experienced sexual abuse was significantly ($p = .02$) associated with a therapist's choice not to touch clients. Therapists who had been sexually abused did tend to touch clients ($p < .02$). And sexual abuse was predictive of whether or not a therapist touched clients, regardless of gender.

In all, 37 therapists (44%) reported sexual abuse. Of these, 28 (76%) of those therapists reporting sexual abuse touched their clients, while 9 (24%) did not touch clients. Forty-seven (56%) of the therapists reported no sexual abuse. Of these therapists, 24 (51%) did not touch clients and 23 (49%) did touch clients. The numbers thus show that almost half of the therapists who reported no sexual abuse touched their clients, while 80% of the therapists who did report sexual abuse touched their clients.

The therapists were also asked whether a teacher or supervisor had ever been sexual with them, and, if so, whether they found the experience to be positive or negative. Thirteen therapists (9 women, 4 men) said that a teacher or supervisor had been sexual with them. Eleven of the therapists found the experience to be negative; only 2 found it positive (1 woman, 1 man). Seven of the therapists (3 men, 4 women) who found the experience to be negative did not touch their clients. The four others (all women) who found the experience to be negative did touch their clients. The two therapists who found the experience to be positive both touched their clients. These therapists both reported that they had also been abused (the man physically; the woman physically and sexually) as children. Two of the male and one of the female therapists did not report the negative sexual experience with a teacher or supervisor on the question that asked about sexual abuse as an adult.

Four female and two male therapists reported that the teacher or supervisor who was sexual with them was also their therapist. All of these experiences were reported as negative. Of these six respondents, the two male therapists and three of the female therapists reported that they did not touch their clients. The remaining female therapist did touch her clients.

No statistical association was found between sexual experiences with therapists/teachers/supervisors and the therapists' practice of touching or not touching their clients. As noted above, about half of the therapists abused by teachers/supervisors/therapists touched their clients in nonerotic ways and half did not.

EFFECTS OF PRESENCE OR ABSENCE OF ABUSE HISTORY ON FEELINGS ABOUT TOUCH

Therapists who reported abuse were asked what effect it had on how they felt about their bodies and about touching and being touched. A frequent response to this question was that the abuse caused them to be sensitive and aware of the impact of touch on others. Here are two typical replies: "It [physical and sexual abuse] made me very sensitive and aware of the impact of touch on others." "I am more sensitive to people who have been abused. I can feel empathy for them. I am more careful about my boundaries and others.' " They also mentioned how the abuse influenced their touching of clients. Here are three examples: "The sex abuse affected how I see the effect of power in relationships and how I use touch in my own therapy with clients." "I had to work through being a clear person to be able to touch [clients]. I hesitate to touch and I'm more careful because of my experience." "Being touched in nonabusive ways [in my own therapy] was very healing for me. So now I touch others because I think it is healing."

The responses given by therapists who reported no sexual abuse and said they touched clients only at greeting, parting or termination fell into two categories. The most often mentioned reason for not touching clients was theoretical. Their theoretical orientation prohibited touch and considered it to be detrimental or not needed for successful treatment. Fears that touch would be misinterpreted, would sexually stimulate clients, would be invasive, would be legally unsafe, or would be unsafe for clients were mentioned. One person cited no training as a reason for not touching. Typical responses included the following: "I don't touch because I'm more concerned about transference misunderstandings: I don't want to open a can of worms." "To touch those with an abuse/trauma history would be an incredible invasion and totally disrupt the therapeutic process. I tell clients their job is to learn to talk about their needs and wishes. Touch would make the therapeutic process an unsafe environment. Touching clients isn't psychotherapy, at least not the way I was taught."

The other category of response related to personal reasons. Several therapists mentioned being personally uncomfortable with the idea of touching clients, as in these examples: "I'm personally not comfortable with touching; it's too complex to analyze." "I was uncomfortable with clients' desire for touch and ambivalent. The result was a firmer adherence to my choice to eliminate touch as a form of therapy."

The same two categories of response were also cited by the therapists who reported no sexual abuse and said that they touched clients. Theoretical orientation and training were mentioned by several therapists as the reason they touched clients. "I feel theoretically supported in touching by my Gestalt, Reichian, bioenergetic orientation. Experientially, I have found it to be helpful to me. I feel comfortable with what I do, and I don't see myself at risk."

The other category, which included the majority of the responses, related to a belief in touching as natural, appropriate, caring, healthy, and healing. These therapists said that touching was comfortable for them, and that they felt they were careful, respectful, and thoughtful about when and why they touched. Typical responses included these: "Touch feels like a natural and appropriate thing to do. It is a natural part of building rapport and being supportive." "Touch is healthy, healing, and natural. It is therapeutic and feels right to do. I'm aware of legal and ethical issues, so I'm careful about boundaries and sex stuff. It doesn't stop me."

INTERACTION BETWEEN PRESENCE OR ABSENCE OF ABUSE HISTORY AND SUBSEQUENT THERAPY/TRAINING EXPERIENCES

After looking at all my data, I noticed that an interaction between a reported history of sexual abuse (or the lack thereof) and subsequent experiences with teachers, supervisors, personal therapists, and training appeared to affect a therapist's choice about touching clients. Two distinct patterns of personal and professional experiences emerged from the data analysis.

Therapists Reporting Sexual Abuse

One pattern of experiences was typical of those therapists who reported having been sexually abused. The abusive experiences with touch seemed to produce both a fear of touch and a hunger for positive, "safe" touch. Safe, positive touch was described as respectful, nurturing, and genuine, and as not sexual, confusing, or unwanted. Since over half of the therapists reporting sexual abuse also reported physical abuse, it was not possible to separate the specific effects of each on the therapist based solely on their responses to open-ended questions. However, the responses to open-ended questions indicated that experiences with abusive touch affected therapists' body image, self-esteem, and feelings about touching and being touched.

The results showed that therapists reporting abuse appeared to seek out experiences to satisfy their need for positive touching. They reported significantly more experiences with body therapies and training in modalities that use touch than did therapists who reported that they were not sexually abused. The therapists would have had to seek out and actively pursue each of these experiences.

The results also showed that therapists with a history of sexual abuse had therapists who touched them. It is not clear from the data how abused therapists came to have therapists who touched them, whereas nonabused therapists had therapists who did not touch them. The responses to the open-ended questions showed that many of the abused therapists found the touching they received from their own therapists to have been very beneficial. Many reported that their experiences with being touched in positive ways in therapeutic situations influenced them to provide similar experiences for their own clients. Perhaps the abused therapists tended to be more likely to touch clients because of awareness of their own needs, past or present, for positive touch.

Therapists with this pattern of experiences were significantly more likely to touch clients. Furthermore, the results suggested that these experiences and resultant beliefs may have influenced therapists to choose a theoretical orientation congruent with their experiences and understanding. The finding, in this study and others (Pope et al., 1987), that therapists with humanistic theoretical orientations are more likely to touch clients, whereas those with psychodynamic theoretical orientations are less likely to touch clients, is consistent with this formulation. More to the point is the finding in my study that therapists who were sexually abused were significantly more likely to subscribe to humanistic theoretical orientations.

Therapists Not Reporting Sexual Abuse

Therapists who did not report experiencing abuse, especially sexual abuse, also did not report indications of touch hunger or say they experienced a need for touch. The responses to the open-ended questions suggested that the nonabused therapists did enjoy touching and being touched in their private lives. Most of the nonabused therapists who did touch clients indicated that they personally enjoyed touching and did it because "I feel like doing it" or "It is a natural extension of my style." And, although they seemed to have healthy and positive beliefs about touch in general, those who chose not to touch clients appeared to have different values and beliefs about touching clients than did those who had experienced sexual abuse. They did not mention sensitivities to and awarenesses of issues related to touch, as therapists who had been abused did. They believed that touch in therapy would stimulate difficult transference issues, and that gratification of touch needs was therapeutically detrimental.

Moreover, therapists who did not report abuse rarely sought out experiences with body therapies, body psychotherapies, or training in modalities involving touch. They were also significantly less likely to have been touched by their own therapists. Therapists with this pattern of experiences were significantly less likely to touch clients, and significantly more likely to report their theoretical orientation as psychodynamic.

A POSSIBLE THIRD PATTERN: AMBIVALENT THERAPISTS

Some therapists reporting that they adhered to a psychodynamic orientation showed ambivalence over the issue of touching clients. Many such therapists reported sexual or physical abuse. The abused therapists tended to touch clients even though they knew it was inconsistent with their theoretical view. Perhaps therapists who have experienced abuse but have not found their way to a theoretical orientation consistent with their experience find that they have diffi-culty adhering to the principles of their orientation.

Comment

The results suggest that therapists who have not been sexually abused may not know what it is like to have been deprived of sufficient "good" touch: touch that is genuine and conveys nurturing, respect, caring, and acceptance. I did not ask therapists about their developmental history: thus, I do not know if any had experienced neglect or other situations which could also produce a developmental deficit of good/safe touch. Nonabused (and not neglected?) therapists seem not to have the same experiential basis for knowing how important touch can be to a person's sense of security, their positive identification with their own bodies, or their basic acceptance of self. The personal experience of therapists who have not been sexually abused differs greatly from those who have been sexually abused and appears to lead therapists to have different kinds of understanding about the value of nonerotic touch in psychotherapy.

THEORETICAL CONSIDERATIONS

Table 6.1 summarizes the differences found in this study between therapists who do and do not touch their clients. The finding that different patterns of experience lead to almost diametrically opposed beliefs and values about the meaning and need for therapeutic touch-ing helps to explain the conflicting theoretical beliefs between the humanistically and psychodynamically oriented about gratification of needs. And it may also explain the lack of consensus, even among some of the humanistically oriented, about whether or not clients who have been sexually abused or have boundary problems should be touched.

The debate among the psychodynamically oriented over whether or not needs should be gratified has a long history. In general, psychoanalytic and psychodynamic theories tend to conclude that gratifying clients' needs for touch is a detrimental therapeutic practice. However, even in the early days of analysis, some were observing that a strict rule of frustration might not always be sufficient. Ferenczi's (1930) inclusion of indulgence as a necessary addition to technique came from noticing that with certain patients, the rule of frustration produced a prolonged (and sometimes unending) mounting of impene-trable resistance. Ferenczi (1930, p. 437) wondered whether the pa-tient's reaction to "a rigid and cold aloofness on the analyst's part" sometimes made the patient suffer more than was absolutely necessary.

TABLE 6.1. Summary of Differences between Therapists Who Touch and Those Who Don't Touch

Therapists who touch	Therapists who don't touch
Usually subscribe to a humanistic theoretical orientation ($p < .01$).	Usually subscribe to a psychodynamic theoretical orientation.
Positively value touch in therapy.	Negatively value touch in therapy.
Believe in touch need/deficit. Believe that gratification of need is therapeutic.	Believe in conflict model; don't believe in deficit model. Believe that gratifying need is detrimental to therapy.
Had therapist(s) who touched them, and found this beneficial ($p < .0001$).	Did not have therapist(s) who touched them.
Had supervisors and teachers who advocated touch as legitimate practice ($p < .0001$).	Did not have teachers and supervisors who advocated touch as legitimate practice.
Have experienced seven or more body therapies ($p = .005$).	Have experienced fewer than seven body therapies.
Have tried more body-oriented psychotherapies ($p = .002$).	Have tried no or few body-oriented psychotherapies.
Have had more training in therapeutic modalities using touch (51+ hrs) ($p < .0001$).	Have had less training in therapeutic modalities using touch (< 50 hrs).
Tend to be female.	Tend to be male.
Likely to have been sexually abused ($p < .02$).	Not likely to have been sexually abused ($p = .02$).

Since that time, several psychodynamic theorists (Bowlby, 1980; Kohut, 1977; Stern, 1985), seeming to follow Ferenczi's lead, have come to contend that pre-Oedipal pathology is due to reality-based deficits rather than psychodynamic "conflicts." Bowlby (1969) has made it clear that attachment has a physical contact aspect. He hypothesized, and others (Main, 1990) have confirmed, that for children at least, the major affective results of appropriate and welcoming physical availability are psychological soothing and safety. Kohut (1977) proposed the term "developmental deficit" to describe adult pathology that he believed to derive from a lack of certain types of experiences normally received as a child.

Brown (1973) is among humanistic theorists who have focused on advocating gratification. He insists that gratification is a necessary precondition to the activation and resolution of psychic trauma. Brown (1973, p. 113) says that "the healing process centers around providing the patient with real here-and-now satisfaction of previously unmet needs for love and caring attention." Brown's position is the same as that taken by hierarchy-of-needs theorists such as Maslow (1968).

Maslow (1968, p. 153) theorized that certain psychological needs are basic because the deprived person yearns for their gratification persistently; because their deprivation makes the person neurotic; because gratifying them is therapeutic; and because healthy (gratified) people do not show these deficiencies. Theorists like Maslow believe that some people have experienced reality-based deficits and need to experience real, supportive interpersonal relationships to repair the damage of neglect and negative parenting. The practical, clinical implication of this view is that in these instances, gratification is therapeutic and frustration is not. For those with deficit-based pathology, understanding their feelings and motivations may not be enough; it appears that the experience of gratification of heretofore unmet needs for nonerotic touch is especially beneficial.

FINAL THOUGHTS

More often than not, the therapists included in this study were proponents of theoretical beliefs and practices that are in line with Kohut's theoretical concept of developmental deficit, Maslow's hierarchy of basic needs, and Brown's theory of therapy. This finding has certain clinical implications. It implies that therapists believe that certain categories of client psychopathology call for gratification of the need state, and that frustration in these instances can be detrimental to the therapeutic course and perhaps unnecessarily painful to the client. The finding that a therapist's values, beliefs, and even theoretical understandings of psychopathology are influenced to a significant extent by his or her personal experience implies that the choice of therapeutic interventions can also be influenced by this experience. Therapists need to be aware of their own bias so that it does not conflict with a client's therapeutic needs.

The results show that therapists who have been sexually abused describe themselves as having touch needs and as having found touch from their own therapists to be a particularly useful intervention. The literature on sexual abuse, most of which indicates that abused clients should not be touched, clearly needs further exploration.

One last conclusion merits serious consideration. The finding that teachers, supervisors, and therapists have a significant impact on the beliefs, values, and practices of the next generation of therapists suggests that they should consider seriously and carefully what they are passing on. Teachers, supervisors, and therapists need to be aware of their own therapeutic value systems and to realize that their own personal experiences have a significant impact on those values. They need to consider carefully whether their values stem from their own unmet needs, or from their having acknowledged and met those needs.

ACKNOWLEDGMENT

This chapter is based on my doctoral dissertation, submitted in partial fulfillment of the requirements for the PhD degree at The Fielding Institute, Santa Barbara, California, 1992.

REFERENCES

Alagna, F. J., Whitcher, S. J., Fisher, J. D., & Wicas, E. A. (1979). Evaluative reaction to interpersonal touch in a counseling interview. *Journal of Counseling Psychology, 26*(6), 465–472.

Bowlby, J. (1980). *Attachment and loss: Vol. 3. Loss: Sadness and depression.* New York: Basic Books.

Brown, M. (1973). The new body therapies. *Psychotherapy: Theory, Research, and Practice, 10,* 98–11.

Ferenczi, F. (1930). The principle of relaxation and neocatharsis. *International Journal of Psycho-Analysis, 2,* 428–443.

Horner, A. J. (1973). To touch—or not to touch. In E. Hendrik & M. Ruitenbeck (Eds.), *The analytic situation: How patients and therapists communicate.* Chicago: Aldine.

Kohut, H. (1977). *The restoration of the self.* New York: International Universities Press.

Kupfermann, K., & Smaldino, C. (1987). The vitalizing and revitalizing experience of reliability: The place of touch in psychotherapy. *Clinical Social Work Journal, 15*(3), 223–234.

Main, M. (1990). Parental aversion to infant-initiated contact is correlated with the parents' own rejection during childhood: The effects of experience on signals of security with respect to attachment. In K. E. Barnard & T. B. Brazelton (Eds.), *Touch: The foundation of experience.* Madison, CT: International Universities Press.

Maslow, A. (1968). *Toward a psychology of being* (2nd ed.). New York: Van Nostrand Reinhold.

Pope, K. S., Tabachnick, B., & Keith-Spiegel, P. (1987). The beliefs and behaviors of psychologists as therapists. *American Psychologist, 42*(11), 1003–1006.

Prochaska, J. O., & Norcross, J. C. (1983). Contemporary psychotherapists: A national survey of characteristics, practices, orientations, and attitudes. *Psychotherapy: Theory, Research, and Practice, 20*(2), 161–173.

Stern, D. N. (1985). *The interpersonal world of the infant.* New York: Basic Books.

Suiter, R. L., & Goodyear, R. K. (1985). Male and female counselor and client perceptions of four levels of counselor touch. *Journal of Counseling Psychology, 32*(4), 645–648.

7

THERAPISTS' RECALL OF THEIR DECISION-MAKING PROCESSES REGARDING THE USE OF TOUCH IN ONGOING PSYCHOTHERAPY

A Preliminary Study

Pauline Rose Clance
Vicki J. Petras

Touch is a major and complex mode of communication between people. In this chapter, we report on therapists' recall of their use of nonsexual and nonaggressive touch within an ongoing, intensive psychotherapy experience.

Touch in psychotherapy has been shown to be very beneficial for some clients. Horton, Clance, Sterk-Elifson, and Emshoff (1995) and Geib (1982) have presented data suggesting that the use of nonerotic physical touch, when done well, can lead to positive outcomes for clients and can be a very powerful healing factor in the psychotherapy process. Hubble, Noble, and Robinson (1981) found that clients who were touched rated their therapists as more expert than did clients who were not touched. Pattison (1973) found that observers judged clients who had been touched as moving more into self-exploration than clients who had not been touched. Alagna, Whitcher, Fisher, and Wicas (1979) found that clients who were touched rated their counseling experience more positively than clients who were not touched. Ford (1989) gives an excellent presentation of cases in which touch was utilized to evoke emotional memories and facilitate the healing process. He also has an excellent chapter on touch as a mediator between the realm of the psyche and the body.

Although touch can be very helpful for some clients, implementing touch within the psychotherapeutic process should be done with much consideration. McNeely (1987), Geib (1982), and Horton et al. (1995) all emphasize monitoring and processing one's touch interventions with the client, and noting the client's associations, reactions, and feedback. McNeely (1987) provides some excellent case examples of utilizing touch with clients in in-depth therapy. She indicates that touch may be used to amplify and explore the unconscious; to mirror content; to decrease body armoring; and to gratify the patient's need for affection, containment, and parenting. However, she emphasizes that gratifying a patient's sexual needs is destructive and should never be done. She also states that "touch that is motivated by the analyst's need for gratification is never justified, and when it is done amounts to exploitation of the patient" (McNeely, 1987, p. 75). Geib (1982) also found that touch, when not done well, could be problematic. (For specifics, see Chapter 8 of this book.)

Given these types of complex issues, we became very interested in the decision-making process regarding touch in psychotherapy. One of us (Vicki J. Petras) approached this issue from a student's point of view, and the other (Pauline Rose Clance) from the point of views of a therapist working with clients. Clance decides with each of her clients whether or not to use touch. There are some clients she has never touched, but touch has been incredibly important in the therapy work of other clients. Clance also teaches psychotherapy at the university level in a PhD program, and she supervises students in their psychotherapy work at the clinic. She struggles as to how best to teach students to provide good psychotherapy, and, within that context, to help them decide when and how touch can be helpful or detrimental.

STUDY I

We decided that it would be helpful to get some information from practicing psychotherapists as to how they made these decisions. We developed a series of questions and distributed them to therapists whom we knew to be interested in intensive psychotherapy, and who might take the time to answer the questions. These psychotherapists were located in the Southeast and either were enrolled in a postgraduate training program in psychotherapy (n = 8), were psychotherapy supervisors and members of the American Academy of Psychotherapy (n = 2), or were receiving psychotherapy supervision from an American Academy supervisor (n = 1). Clearly, this was not a random sample of therapists in the Southeast; it was a sample of therapists obtained by means of a networking procedure. These are therapists whom we knew by their reputation and interest in psychotherapy, and who were willing to spend an hour or two in answering a very detailed questionnaire. Consequently, the information we gained was from clinicians who were interested enough in psychotherapy to obtain additional training beyond that necessary to get a license, and who had at least 2 years of experience in providing psychotherapy to clients. In addition, most of them had a general practice. The number of years of postgraduate clinical experience of these psychotherapists ranged from 4 to 41, with a mean of 13 years.

Although this was a nonrandom, nonrepresentative sample of psychotherapists, the information received is important, in that it tells us of the self-reports of experienced, interested clinicians on a topic that has not previously been empirically investigated. Clearly, the findings reported here cannot be generalized to all clinicians; nevertheless, they do provide us with significant information on these experienced clinicians' views of their decision-making processes regarding touch within ongoing psychotherapy. The reader can use this information to stimulate his or her thinking on the subject, and can compare his or her own clinical experience to that of these clinicians. In addition, we hope that this information will be helpful to clinical researchers as they begin to study touch within ongoing psychotherapy.

We distributed 35 questionnaires (see Table 7.1) and received 11 replies. (Several nonrespondents spontaneously let us know that they found the questionnaire too hard or too time-consuming. Several others reported that they wanted to talk about the issues because they had great difficulty in writing down the responses.) As Table 7.1 indicates, we asked respondents to describe two clients whom they had touched within ongoing psychotherapy and two clients whom they had not touched. We asked them to describe the history, demographics, and psychological characteristics of each pair of clients.

Lists of the clients described by the 11 respondents as touched and not touched are provided in Tables 7.2 and 7.3, respectively. (Not every respondent listed two clients in each category of touched and not touched.)

A study of these two tables indicates no discernible patterns of

TABLE 7.1. Questionnaire on Touch in Psychotherapy

Dear Colleague,

Edward Smith, Pauline Rose Clance, and Suzanne Imes are editing a book about the use of touch in psychotherapy. We are writing a chapter on therapists' decisions to touch or not to touch particular clients. Will you help us discover some of the ways therapists make these decisions? If so, please write to us about the following information:

I. Take into consideration two clients (Clients 1 and 2) you have touched in psychotherapy. For both clients, indicate the following:
    A. Brief psychological history, how long in therapy, age, sex, race.
    B. How did you decide it would be beneficial to touch this client? What were the particular characteristics and issues of this client that influenced your decision to touch? What benefits did you think touching would have for the client?
    C. In what way(s) did you touch the client (holding, touching particular tension points to release feelings, etc.)?
    D. Do you think touching has been beneficial? How or how not?
    E. (Optional) Did your theoretical orientation to therapy influence your decision to touch this client? If so, how?
II. Take into consideration two clients (Clients 3 and 4) you decided *not to touch* in psychotherapy. For both clients, include the following:
    A. Brief psychological history, how long in therapy, age, sex, race.
    B. How did you decide not to touch this client? What were the particular characteristics and issues of this client that influenced your decision to touch?
    C. Do you think not touching this client has been beneficial?
    D. (Optional) Did your theoretical orientation to therapy influence your decision not to touch this client?

differences between the clients who were touched and those who were not. No significant historical features or diagnostic categories emerged to differentiate the two groups. This is important information. The reports from our respondents suggest that diagnosis and history are not the critical determining variables in the decision to touch or not to touch clients; however, this information is not ignored by therapists and seems to be considered to some extent in their decisions regarding touch. There remains a need for a large-scale empirical study to investigate the role played by diagnosis and history in the decision to touch or not to touch clients.

We asked the respondents to explain how they decided to touch or not to touch clients. Listed in Table 7.4 are the therapists' recollections of reasons for deciding to touch or not to touch. (A respondent could give more than one reason.)

As shown in the table, some of the main reasons why these therapists used touch were to help clients access feelings in a healthy way, to respond to clients' requests to be touched, and to provide a

TABLE 7.2. History and Demographics of Clients Who Were Touched

Males

16 years old; father left after a divorce from his mother
35 years old; Caucasian; divorced; alcoholic
40 years old; Caucasian; suffers from a diffuse pain
Late 40s; married; psychologically abused and rejected by his father; low
  self-esteem and very self-critical
Caucasian; severe obsessive–compulsive disorder; grew up in a chaotic,
  uproarious family
Seven males in an HIV+ group; all functioning well psychologically; dealing
  with a physical illness

Females

24 years old; abandoned by her mother
25 years old; Caucasian; features of obsessive–compulsive disorder;
  hospitalized for bulimia nervosa in college
25 years old; needed help with a significant decision
26 years old; Caucasian; major depression; history of psychiatric hospitalizations
35 years old; married, mother; husband diagnosed with terminal cancer
Late 30s; Caucasian; atypical dissociative disorder
Late 30s; Caucasian; severe obsessive–compulsive symptoms; extensive history
  of physical and emotional abuse
40 years old; severely beaten by her mother
40 years old; emotional and weepy; unsatisfactory relationships
40 years old; Caucasian; married; extensive psychiatric history; dissociative
  identity disorder
42 years old; Caucasian; divorced; anxiety and depression; difficulty with
  relationships; trust and abandonment issues
42 years old; African-American; physically, emotionally, and sexually abused
  by father
40 years old; Caucasian; deals with considerable depression and anxiety; some
  self-destructiveness in her 20s; white-collar professional with master's degree
40 years old; Caucasian; single; sexually abused by her father; no expression
  of feelings; family was very sarcastic
Caucasian; incipient schizophrenia; severe disturbances
Caucasian; domineering and cruel father; separated from mother for 3 days
  after birth
Abuse history; few to no dissociative processes; good reality testing and able
  to check out any misconceptions as they occur
Felt dirty and untouchable; history of abuse; no dissociative processes

model for safe and nurturing touch. The first of these findings (i.e., that touch helped clients to access feelings in a healthy way) is similar to that of Pattison's (1973) study, in which observers judged clients who had been touched as moving more into self-exploration than clients who had not been touched. On the other hand, therapists suggested that some of the main reasons why they would not touch particular

TABLE 7.3. History and Demographics of Clients Who Were Not Touched

Males

Teenager; Caucasian; head injury

26 years old; Caucasian; sexual addiction; verbally abusive and distant father

30 years old; Hispanic; posttraumatic stress disorder; flashbacks after being beaten in jail cell

34 years old; sexual abuse history; lacked sufficient boundaries in interpersonal relationships

37 years old; relationship difficulties and stated he had no boundaries with women

38 years old; Caucasian; single, artistic, and gentle; teased mercilessly as a child about playing with girls; reclusive, few friends, few interests; can't sustain relationships with women

Elderly Caucasian; full of ailments and complaints; chronically unhappy; frozen in his emotions

Professional with history of sexual misconduct

Females

18 years old; Caucasian; felt some sexual attraction; flirtation on her part

26 years old; Caucasian; history of destructive relationships, substance abuse; psychiatric hospitalization

27 years old; Caucasian; extensive history of very severe sexual and physical abuse; dissociation and posttraumatic stress disorder; depressed and self-destructive

Late 30s; African-American; single mother; works full-time, no child support; two children

Late 30s; Caucasian; agoraphobic and dissociative; vague memories of sexual abuse

42 years old; Caucasian; bipolar; drug and alcohol history; extensive psychotic hospitalizations; emotional, physical, and sexual abuse

47 years old; divorced; overeating; sexual abuse by father

50 years old; Caucasian; divorced; ex-spouse sexually abused child; father abusive to mother

56 years old; African-American; schizophrenic; psychotic episodes; tended to merge with people

Caucasian; psychotic core; illusions and delusions; paranoid thought disorder and with her psychotic process would misinterpret events; sexual abuse survivor; frequently told me she loved me and stared at me intently

clients was that touch could have been easily misinterpreted by the clients and that touch could have been too intense and invasive during that point of the therapeutic process.

Table 7.5 is a list of therapists' responses concerning the benefits of touching versus not touching their clients.

The respondents clearly perceived both touching and not touching as having clear benefits in various contexts. As shown in the table,

TABLE 7.4. Therapists' Reasons for Deciding to Touch or Not to Touch

Reason	n
Reasons for deciding to touch	
Helped to access feelings in a healthy way	7
Client asked to be touched or hugged	6
A model for safe and nurturing touch	5
History of touch deprivation	4
Touch in previous therapy seemed helpful to the client	3
To give comfort and support	2
Good-bye hug at termination	1
Good ego strength and coping skills and touch seemed helpful	1
Reasons for deciding not to touch	
Could be easily misinterpreted due to clients' issues surrounding touch (e.g., not good boundaries, might seem disrespectful, sexual connotation)	4
Too intense and invasive at that point in therapy	3
Client able to access feelings without touch	1
Attraction between client and therapist	1
Touch had no meaning for the client	1
Client needed structure of clear boundaries	1
Touch was unbearable for client	1

therapists thought that one of the main benefits of touch in psychotherapy was that it increased trust and safety both within and outside of therapy. On the other hand, therapists reported that some of the main benefits of not touching were that it kept boundaries defined or clear and enhanced clients' feelings of safety and control. Thus, in their subjective judgment and experience, these therapists saw touch as increasing safety and trust for one set of clients, whereas *not* touching was seen as enhancing safety and trust for another set. As we read the

TABLE 7.5. Therapists' Perceptions of Benefits of Touching versus Not Touching Clients

Benefits of touching clients	
Increased trust and safety within therapy and outside of therapy	10
Helped client experience/release feelings	7
Enabled client to experience nurturing and safe touch with others	2
Benefits of not touching clients	
Kept boundaries defined/clear	7
Enhanced clients' feelings of safety and control	7
Pushed client to experience his or her pain and strengths without touch	2
Had no relevance to therapy work	1

questionnaire responses from these therapists in their entirety, it seemed that the needs of the clients, as seen by the therapists, were the primary factors influencing their decision to touch or not to touch.

We were curious as to how much therapists saw their theoretical orientation as affecting their decision to touch or not to touch. We made this an optional question. Of the 11 respondents, 7 stated that their theoretical orientation definitely influenced their decision to utilize touch within psychotherapy. One respondent was unsure about the role of theoretical orientation, and one stated that theoretical orientation was not important. Only 6 of the 11 respondents answered the question regarding the role of their theoretical orientation in deciding not to touch. It may be that the question seemed too repetitious and that it was the last question, so that respondents simply gave it less energy. Four respondents indicated their theoretical orientation affected their decision not to touch, and two stated that it did not. Still, theoretical orientation was a variable that was considered by over 50% of these clinicians when deciding to touch or not to touch.

STUDY 2

In an effort to get a larger number of respondents, we changed the questionnaire and made it simpler and less time-consuming (see Table 7.6). Then we sent this new questionnaire to approximately 20 different therapists who were in advanced training in psychotherapy, were members of the American Academy of Psychotherapy, or were psychotherapy supervisors. The number of years of postgraduate clinical experience of these psychotherapists ranged between 2 and 27, with a mean of 9 years. We received 11 responses and found the responses interesting and informative. As we have stated earlier in regard to Study

TABLE 7.6. Revised Questionnaire on Touch in Psychotherapy

Dear Psychotherapist,

    Please help us understand your decision process concerning when to touch and when not to touch clients. Please think of two clients whom you have decided not to touch in psychotherapy, and two clients for whom you have used touch in your treatment.

    Please describe how you decided to touch and not to touch. How are the clients you did not touch different from the clients you did touch in therapy? What stands out to you as the main difference between clients? Also, please describe your decision-making process in one or two paragraphs.

    Thank you so much for your help.

1, these responses were nonrandom and are not representative of clinicians in general, but do give us information from experienced practicing psychotherapists with a strong interest and experience in doing psychotherapy. To eliminate redundancy, we have chosen not to present all of the responses here. The following eight responses each describe different decision-making processes in regard to using or not using touch in psychotherapy. When clients are discussed, names and identifying information have been changed to protect their privacy or a composite of several clients was used when indicated.

RESPONSE 1

I have touched clients minimally in my work. I am very careful with touch, but particularly cautious when a client has any history of sexual abuse. I've had two female adult clients with that history who have initiated physical contact: hugging in one, wanting to crawl in my lap in the other. In the first case, with a new client I received the hug but did not return it. This client also had difficulty with limiting the session to 50 minutes. I handled it all by apologizing (at the beginning of the next session) for not minding the time boundary carefully enough. Therapy has gone smoothly since then. In the second client situation, she wanted to regress at a time when it seemed particularly important that she learn to be more adult. We discussed this, and her work evolved into maintaining intimate contact with a minimum of touching (I put my arm around her). There were a couple of situations where I wrapped a blanket around her or helped her to feel her physical boundary and containment on her own.

On the other hand, I would return a hug initiated by a client upon termination or by a client who has a clear sense of her physical self (and no history of abuse). I will also shake hands when initiated by the client.

RESPONSE 2

Generally, if I am feeling inclined to make physical contact with a client, I will share/talk about my sense of responsiveness to the client and will ask if my initiating contact fits with what the client is needing at the time. I will not make contact with a client unless I know it is what the client wants.

The clients I do not initiate physical contact with are those who have some history of boundary violation (i.e., physical, sexual, emotional abuse) and/or have a tendency to oversexualize or be seductive, and/or have compromised/poorly differentiated ego boundaries. If, however, these clients initiate contact with me, I do not reject their contact (unless it is really inappropriate . . . this has never been the case for me, however). I do explore the meaning of the contact and process my own or the clients' reactions.

It seems, for me, that the main difference between clients I initiate physical contact with and those I do not initiate contact with is the clients' level of ego functioning or sense of boundaries—the lower the ego functioning, the less inclined I am to initiate contact.

RESPONSE 3

Because I am a Latina, the issue of touch in psychotherapy for me is intricately intertwined with ethnicity—mine and the client's. Two clients I have touched in therapy have both been Latinos, and the idea of not touching in therapy would have been quite foreign and would undoubtedly be perceived as cold, distant, and uncaring. One was a man from a South American country in his mid-30s, who had been depressed for a long time. I was the first Spanish-speaking therapist he had had in this country, and he was relieved that he would be able to be understood in the subtle ways that a second language does not allow. He extended his hand in greeting at the very beginning of the first session. I of course followed suit—to do otherwise would have been unthinkable. I suspect the first session would also have been the last. At the end of that session he asked for a hug, which I gave him. I remembered thinking how well we seemed to have connected in such a short time—the request for a hug told me he felt good about our session. I had a shock as I presented the session to my Anglo supervisor: She took a completely different view of the hug, and asked me to look deeply into myself and try to find the real reason for my agreeing to hug my client. She saw it as a breach of boundaries and a dangerous first step in our therapeutic relationship. My attempt at explaining the meaning of touch in our culture (mine and the client's!) was minimized and dismissed.

Another client I have touched in therapy is more of a composite of many Latinas with whom I have worked. She was a Mexican woman in her 20s, and she came to me because she was being abused by her husband. As is customary in our culture between women, I touched her arm or her shoulder (rather than shaking her hand) when she first came in, put my hand on her arm when she cried, and hugged her at the end of each session (she did not need to ask for this verbally—I am Latina and she was expecting it).

When I am working with Latino clients, the issue of touch in therapy becomes more part of the context of therapy, as opposed to a tool I would use in certain cases. The same does not hold true for my work with Anglo and African-American clients. One of the clients I decided not to touch (for the first 10 months of therapy or so) was an African-American man in his 40s, a recovering heroin addict who was also HIV+. He was quite distrustful of the whole system, myself included, and it was clear from the way he carried himself and the distance he moved his chair away from mine that he needed plenty of personal space. I remember making a mental note of these details and actively deciding at the end of the session not to touch him. (I remember feeling unsure if he would come back for subsequent sessions. Both his addiction history and the distance he kept from me made me doubtful. I was surprised and delighted when he continued coming to our weekly sessions.) After almost a year of therapy, on his birthday I asked him if I could give him a birthday hug. He was both surprised and very pleased. Since that time, this has become our parting ritual. His chair is a lot closer to mine now, and his body appears much more open.

The other client whom I decided not to touch was an Anglo woman in her early 20s, a graduate student who was also depressed. Despite her apparent sophistication regarding therapy and eagerness to be involved in the process, I sensed her need to be a private person, and in her case, her need for physical distance. I remember thinking I would let her take the lead, and I would follow it. I believe I was concerned about invading her space, and I wanted to be very respectful of this issue. At the end of our time together (about 12 sessions, I was finishing my internship), she still appeared to me to prefer keeping her distance. I followed her lead.

Although it would appear that ethnicity would be the variable that would affect my decision to touch or not in therapy, the issue for me is more complex. As a feminist therapist, I am always aware of my power status vis-à-vis my clients. I think that touch in therapy at times can serve (as well as other things, of course) as an equalizing factor in our relationship. Touch is also something that comes to me naturally—something I will use with my clients (regardless of ethnicity) unless I perceive that their need for space, distance, or the like precludes my touching them.

The difference between the Anglo and African-American clients I have touched or not seems to be my perception of their need for personal space and their body language. Although I have not yet had a Latino client I have not touched, I would hope that my "ethnic blinders" would not prevent me from being aware of this special need in any of them, and from honoring this need, regardless of our common ethnic scripts.

RESPONSE 4

Essentially, I offer touch, provide touch in response to a request for it, or provide spontaneous touch to clients who are emotionally available and vulnerable to themselves and to me. I will provide touch as a means of emotional comfort, affirmation of the client, and affirmation of the value of the therapist–client relationship. Factors that help me decide whom I touch versus whom I don't touch include the following: (1) the duration of the therapy, so the longer I work with someone, the more likely I am to provide touch; (2) the client's expressed and/or demonstrated comfort (e.g., client sits closer to therapist rather than farther away) in the therapist–client relationship; (3) perception of a client's ability to approach issues of transference in a healthy manner (i.e., to process relational issues within the context of the therapist–client relationship); and (4) the nature of the client's work, so that touch, in some instances, seems more appropriate for clients who generally engage in in-depth self-exploration than for those who generally pursue immediate problem solving. The main difference between whom I touch in therapy and whom I don't is, perhaps, that the former more than the latter appear more willing to take risks in their strivings for fuller emotional and relational functioning with themselves and with others.

RESPONSE 5

I do not think of touch I have with clients as part of treatment, though I suppose it could be seen as such, in that it is part of the interaction. The touching I do ranges from a minimum of no touch at all to a maximum of a hug at the end of the session. I never use touch during sessions. My therapy is eclectic, but would best be characterized as a blend of Rogerian, psychodynamic, and cognitive. I am very aware of and respectful of boundaries as part of my personality, as well as part of my theoretical beliefs. I don't do regressive work to any large degree and do not foster dependence, though I try to pay attention to transference and countertransference. If someone wanted some form of touch during a session (e.g., to be held), I would probably try to validate the wish and help them understand the need, but decline to do it, explaining that it would make me uncomfortable because of who I am as a person and as a therapist (i.e., taking responsibility for my own feelings and trying hard not to shame them or make them feel rejected).

Regarding the touch that I do use at the start and end of sessions, I take my cues from the client. Typically, I shake hands with both male and female clients when I meet them, unless they convey through body language that it might be experienced as intrusive (I am a male, by the way). With female clients, I typically would not shake hands in subsequent sessions unless they initiate it. With male clients, I frequently shake hands at the end of all sessions, since that behavior is socially accepted and usually comfortable male behavior. I rarely initiate hugs at the end of sessions, though I find that maybe 30%–40% of my clients initiate hugs at the end. I am very responsive and pleased to give them this physical support if they initiate it. I don't initiate hugs because I believe they could make many clients uncomfortable and be experienced as intrusive. An additional form of touch I sometimes use, whether a hug or handshake has occurred or not, is to gently place my hand on their back for a moment as they leave, if their body cues indicate that they are open to this and would welcome the support.

RESPONSE 6

Both of the clients whom I decided not to touch had histories of physical and sexual abuse. Their nonverbal communication and body language seemed rather closed, and I felt that it was important to allow them to modulate their degree of comfort with touch.

The clients I have touched have been more open, in that they make eye contact more freely and for longer periods and have typically displayed some degree of mirroring of my body language (e.g., leaning in when I lean in, standing more in closer proximity to me when leaving).

Interestingly, the two clients with whom I have used touch (usually a hug good-bye or a pat on the arm) also had histories of abuse. This realization makes me think that I am relying more on nonverbal cues than on my knowledge or theoretical notions about what might be appropriate for them.

RESPONSE 7

When I think about using therapeutic touch, I think it's important to recognize the power of touch and the potential for multilayered communication afforded by its use. Thus, it's important to me to be very conscious about my decisions concerning when and when not to touch, while balancing that consciousness with a "realness" or degree of spontaneity. I think of several issues when considering touch—including client dynamics, my comfort, and the client's comfort—all interacting in complex ways. Regarding client dynamics, I consider the role of touch in the client's history; the meaning of touch to the client (e.g., nurturing, intruding, etc.); history of sexual or physical abuse; ego strength; psychological boundaries; and so forth. I consider the complex interplay of such issues in formulating a decision about how to use touch, and I don't believe that there are rigid or set answers, but rather believe that the unique constellations of issues in my client and in our interaction inform my decisions. For example, a history of sexual abuse might contraindicate touch, especially in combination with compromised psychological boundaries and a construction of meaning that touch is equal to victimization or intrusion. However, for another client, nonsexual, safe touch, regulated by the client (with responsibility for limits on the therapist), may serve as a corrective, healing experience. If I try to identify any set parameters, I can only think of the following: (1) I would not touch a client who expresses a desire not to be touched; (2) I won't touch if I'm uncomfortable, as I assume my comfort level to be a source of information; and (3) the primary rule of touch—never, ever engage in sexualized touch with a client. Beyond those, I evaluate client dynamics in making a decision.

Regarding clients whom I would or would not touch, I can only consider people I've worked with. I have chosen not to touch clients who have expressed confusion or lack of clarity around their ownership of their bodies and their abilities to set psychological or physical limits. I assume in all cases that I will be responsible for limits around safety, and where notable confusion regarding limits in the client is primary, I will make this responsibility explicit in order to provide a safe container of sorts wherein such issues can be explored freely.

Clients I have touched are those who tend to be somewhat disconnected, often in a manner that actively pushes others away or in a manner that is marked by lack of warmth and loneliness. With those clients, I have been careful first to develop a solid therapeutic relationship (without touch) and then only later to incorporate small, brief (but warm) touches (e.g., when leaving the office). My hope in this is to communicate via multiple channels my availability, acceptance, and consistency for the client.

I think that, in general, I use touch sparingly. I am aware of its power, and I am aware of the inherent power differential in the therapeutic relationship. I believe in recognizing this differential while striving to equalize as much as is possible by respecting the dignity of my clients. As such, I try to remain aware of the empowerment of my clients and strive never to infantilize or disempower. Just as touch has tremendous healing potential, I also believe it can be powerfully used in destructive ways. Thus I am careful (and rather conservative) in my use of touch. So my touch tends, in most cases, to involve a light touch on the shoulder or arm, a hand held during moments of grief, or an occasional good-bye hug (most often client-initiated). Where I think touch might confuse or upset—rather than calm or clarify—I tend not to touch at all. It's difficult to make explicit so complex a decision in a few paragraphs. But I've tried here to capture the essence of my clinical thinking on this issue.

RESPONSE 8

[Note: All patient names in this response are pseudonyms.]
Physical touch is not a regular part of my therapy, with the

following exceptions. I often greet both new and continuing clients in the waiting room with a handshake. I walk all clients to the door following the session, and sometimes shake hands as a "Well done" or a "Go well" gesture. I may also touch a shoulder or arm in a similar way.

Examples of touching:

(1) I hugged Joanne (age 70; I'm 58) as she left the session. I meet her monthly, pretty much on a supportive basis. She has had much on her mind, which she tries not to burden her family with. She's a strong woman, but life is difficult. I think we both understood the hug as affirmation of the tough times, of my care for her, and of my confidence in her. It was a "Carry on" hug. I didn't think much about it—it simply was not contraindicated. It would not interfere with our working relationship.

(2) I had been meeting with Mary (age 54) twice a month, to help her deal with alcohol problems, a dying mother, and the end of a 15-year relationship with a lover. Early in our work she held herself aloof, despite efforts to appear casual and to erase thera-pist–client lines. She proclaimed that she knows how to be cool-headed as the situation demands. She often sidestepped my urgings that she confront various issues. On several occasions in those early sessions, I allowed myself to tap her Reebok (her leg crossed at knee) with my hand, surprising her with that unortho-dox indication that she should return to the issue. My reasoning was that it was a quick, direct way to cut through avoidance, bypassing discussions and power struggles. I think that my tap suited her insistence on being laid back and casual, while allowing me to insist on doing our work.

(3) This third example fills out the sample. Tara was in her mid-20s, a survivor of sexual and other abuse throughout child-hood. She was bright and lively, but fragmented and dissociative. Well into our first year, after I had gotten to know several "personalities," I found that the tough, angry, cold one both held the rest together and intimidated them. In one session I instructed that they should all stay in the room at the same time, instead of flitting in and out, so we'd all have the same information. When "tough Tara" got up and paced around my office, moving books, vases, and other objects around impetuously, I somehow knew that she was in touch with being all these vulnerable selves. I knew that she was showing me that she couldn't find a way to settle in, was frightened, and so on. I stood up, intercepted her, and embraced her—at first to contain her, and then to "hold" her in Winnicott's sense. At first stiff, she relaxed and calmed; we stood that way for about 3 minutes. My rationale was that I could reach her at that

moment in a reparative, transformative way that words alone would never manage. That day was a turning point, a grounding for many years of work to come—work that finally concluded with an integrated Tara.

Examples of not touching:

(1) I walk well behind Jerry (age 45), who has attempted to encircle my waist for lingering seconds as he leaves the session. I now avoid even a handshake, which he has turned into a gliding farewell. Rationale: I want him to come to know that I won't let him live out a long-term pattern with me. By my disallowing his habitual inclination (flirting under the guise of sincerity), I hope that he also will become more aware of the inclination on his own. At that point, the doorway dynamics may be useful for discussion.

(2) Ellie (in her 40s) expends considerable effort in our sessions to elicit sympathy, encouragement, and rescuing. In an effort to counter what I experience as her pulling for me to comfort her physically as she leaves, I instead walk well behind her to the exit door. I smile and warmly remind her of her therapy "homework" for the week. Recently, at the door she beat me to saying what the homework was. We later discussed her discovering that she can receive support and care without having to be "taken care of."

So I guess I employ touching and not touching to communicate beyond words at the moment. Not touching often reminds clients and me that this is not an ordinary social relationship, but rather a work relationship, even though between two people in a particular kind of intimacy. Not responding physically to pulls for touch helps both parties to become more aware of the pull and to wonder about its place in the client's life in and out of therapy.

Some clients hold themselves back from even a potential handshake, and that's fine with me. I accommodate to family and personal traditions. I don't think much in terms of diagnostic categories in regard to touching. Rather, I think more in terms of developmental level, and what would likely be the meaning to the person I touch.

In summary, these therapists clearly put much thought into their decisions to touch or not to touch clients. Many variables, such as the clients' ego strength, dynamics, needs, body language and cues, history regarding touch, length of time in therapy, and others, might affect their decisions with particular clients. The response from the Latina therapist (Response 3) is important in highlighting the importance of cultural norms regarding touch. The therapists used their own thinking and judgment about clients in the decisions they described, rather than a rule to touch or not to touch. They seemed to give thoughtful consideration to the individual clients as they made their decisions. This type of processing by therapists regarding any decision in therapy seems important.

REFERENCES

Alagna, F. J., Whitcher, S. J., Fisher, J. D., & Wicas, E. A. (1979). Evaluative reaction to interpersonal touch in a counseling interview. *Journal of Counseling Psychology, 26,* 465–472.

Ford, C. (1989). *Where healing waters meet: Touching mind and emotion through body.* Tarrytown, NY: Station Hill Press.

Geib, P. (1982). The experience of nonerotic contact in traditional psychotherapy: A critical investigation of the taboo against touch. *Dissertation Abstracts International, 43,* 113A.

Horton, J. A., Clance, P. R., Sterk-Elifson, C., & Emshoff, J. (1995). Touch in psychotherapy: A survey of patients' experiences. *Psychotherapy, 32,* 443–457.

Hubble, M. A., Noble, F. C., & Robinson, S. E. (1981). The effect of counselor touch in an initial counseling session. *Journal of Counseling Psychology, 28,* 533–535.

McNeely, D. A. (1987). *Touching: Body therapy and depth psychology.* Toronto: Inner City Books.

Pattison, J. E. (1973). Effects of touch on self exploration and the therapeutic relationship. *Journal of Consulting and Clinical Psychology, 40,* 170–175.

THE EXPERIENCE OF NONEROTIC PHYSICAL CONTACT IN TRADITIONAL PSYCHOTHERAPY

Pamela Geib

THE BACKGROUND FOR THIS RESEARCH

When I told people that I was studying nonerotic physical contact, many of them would give me a knowing look and say, "There's no such thing as *nonerotic* physical contact!" This made for many exciting conversations, and it also revealed in some way the heart of the issue: how hard it is for many people to differentiate between sex and other types of physical contact. This is a general difficulty in our culture, but it is especially difficult and highly charged in the field of psychotherapy. There is no particular controversy surrounding, say, the intimacies of a dentist who puts fingers (or sometimes a whole hand) in a patient's mouth; but in psychotherapy, it's a different story.

The power of the controversy regarding touch in therapy results in part from the paradox that *is* therapy: a relationship that is profound, intimate, and intense on the one hand, and formal, professional, and well-bounded on the other. Our job as therapists is to stay close, but to stay clear—clear about what we're doing, and clear in communicating limits and boundaries. In some way, one could say that we are to love, and to love professionally: an informed, thoughtful, yet heart-felt connection. Given the complexities and power of the therapeutic relationship, it is no wonder that touch is a difficult subject—no wonder that it has been traditionally prohibited in order that boundaries stay clear, and that sexual abuse not take place.

And prohibited it has been. Freud, who initially placed his hands on the foreheads of patients to facilitate free association, came later to repudiate vociferously any physical contact. He made this abundantly clear in a letter to Sandor Ferenczi (see Chapter 1, p. 8). Ferenczi had begun experimenting in his own work with patients. Rather than solely interpreting the needs of patients, he began in some cases to gratify their expressions of need. This technique, which he called "the principle of relaxation," sometimes included the physical holding of patients. Freud responded to this news with a rather hysterical letter indicating that he equated physical contact with sex: Why stop, he asked Ferenczi, at holding? "Certainly one gets further when one adopts pawing as well. And then bolder ones will come along who will go further to peeping and showing and soon we will have petting parties, resulting in an enormous increase of interest in psychoanalysis among both analysts and patients" (quoted in Jones, 1955, p. 163).

More recently, Karl Menninger (1958, p. 40) stated: "Transgression of the rule against physical contact constitutes evidence of the incompetence or criminal ruthlessness of the analyst." And a contemporary of Menninger's, the psychiatrist L. R. Wolberg (1954, p. 606), wrote: "It goes without saying that physical contact with patients is absolutely taboo."

This taboo was and is meant to insure the safety of the client, but it raises several problems. First, it does prevent some therapists from making use of touch. Yet my research shows that touch can be a powerful healing force when used appropriately. Second, this taboo does not prevent many other therapists from sometimes touching their clients, but it does often make them feel guilty and secretive about their behavior. So the subject is not discussed with supervisors or colleagues.

Surveys conducted in 1969 (Forer, 1969, p. 230) and in 1977 (Holroyd & Brodsky, 1977; cited in Tyson, 1979) demonstrated that over 50% of therapists in two large anonymous samples did make selective use of physical contact in their work. Yet clinicians are reluctant to discuss this aspect their work openly. Jules Older (1977) illustrated this point in recounting a supervision experience with a young psychiatrist who had just seen a very difficult patient. As he listened to an account of the session, Older suggested that this was a case in which the therapist might have appropriately touched the client. The supervisee admitted sheepishly that he had in fact held the patient during the session, but that he'd been afraid to bring it up in supervision. After this experience, Older interviewed many therapists who said they felt comfortable with the use of physical contact when appropriate. Many of these same people, though, did not feel at all comfortable in discussing such contact with colleagues or supervisors.

One of the most interesting examples of the importance of opening up this topic for examination is given in a paper by Merle Jordan (1970), entitled "Supervision of a Defensive Non-Verbal Communication." Jordan described a supervision in which the supervisee felt that he was being supportive and warm by responding positively to a client's request to hold her hand sometimes during the session. Jordan discovered that the hand holding took place only when it would have been more appropriate for the client to be angry. He saw the contact as a way in which the client and therapist were colluding to avoid communicating about anger. Through supervision, the defensive nature of the touching was understood. Had it gone unreported, the entire nature of the therapeutic process might have remained a puzzle to both supervisor and therapist. And it often does go unreported.

Again, I had some personal experience of this when I was doing my research. Word got around the clinic where I worked that my topic was touch. I found myself ambushed in corridors and dragged off to offices, where staff members "confessed" that "There was this special time when . . . ," "It happened that there was this unusual circumstance . . . ," "I had this distraught client . . . ," and so on. I was hearing that there had been many instances in which therapists had been moved to touch clients, but had been afraid to discuss, and therefore unable to evaluate, this contact.

We are talking, then, about touch in therapy—something that happens a fair amount; that is talked about very little; that is surrounded by strong fears and prohibitions because of its link with sexuality; *and* that has an extremely charged meaning in this powerful context of psychotherapy, in which the therapist is both an intimate and yet professional other. The context of psychotherapy is further charged by current realities that make an examination of the use of touch even more complex and more salient. Two important factors inform this current context: (1) our increasing knowledge of and concern about actual sexual abuse of clients by therapists; and (2) the increasing numbers of clients who know themselves to be adult survivors of childhood sexual abuse.

The first factor—our increasing awareness of sexual abuse in the therapeutic situation—serves an extremely positive function. It sharpens our awareness of the distress that any boundary violation, most especially a sexual one, causes clients. We hope that clients are safer because of this recent publicity. But our awareness has a problematic facet as well. The fear of being misunderstood by their clients can inhibit therapists who might otherwise use touch to good effect. In addition, the fear of being misunderstood by colleagues and the fear of lawsuits may deepen the silence around this topic; thus, essential opportunities for supervision and thoughtful scrutiny may be lost.

The second factor—the increasing numbers of clients who are coming to know that they are survivors of childhood sexual abuse—loads the issue of touch in another way. Working with people who have been violated through physical contact requires strict observance of boundaries, both emotional and physical. Paradoxically but understandably, some of the clients who are working through issues of sexual abuse are the very ones who sometimes request and even demand that a holding environment be made concrete: They wish to be held physically in order to better bear their pain.

Having emphasized how important I believe this subject is, I'd like to discuss the development of my own views about touch in psychotherapy. What drew my attention to the subject of physical contact was my interest in the object relations school of therapy. Object relations emphasizes the pre-Oedipal issues concerned with very early mother–child interactions. It looks specifically at the role of nurturance and empathy both in the early history of the patient and in the therapeutic relationship. My contention is that within such a framework, it becomes possible to speak of *nonerotic* touch. Within the traditional psychoanalytic framework, which is Oedipal and drive-oriented, touch is seen as essentially sexual. But within the framework of an individual's need for nurturance and support, touch can be viewed as both essential and nonerotic, although sexual overtones can obviously exist.

D. W. Winnicott (1958), a famous object relations theorist, wrote of how therapists could create a "holding environment," in which patients who had not had adequate or "good enough" mothering at an early age could be "held" through long periods of regression. Winnicott (quoted by Kahn in the foreword to Winnicott, 1975, p. xxvi) defined the holding environment as "The quality of setting in which the patient is free from environmental impingement and the provision by the analyst of what is required by the patient: be it abstention from intrusion by interpretation, and/or a sensitive body-presence in his person, and/or letting the patient move around and just be and do what he needs to." He also poignantly wrote (quoted by Kahn in Winnicott, 1975, p. xxix): "The behavior of the analyst, by being 'good enough' in the matter of adaptation to need, is gradually perceived by the patient as something that raises the hope that the true self may at last be able to take the risks involved in its starting to experience living."

When I read Winnicott, I was very much moved by his description of therapy, but I also began to realize that I didn't really know what he meant by a "holding environment." Obviously, he meant some kind of empathic resonating with the experience of the patient. He also meant a willingness on the part of the therapist to recreate, in some manner, the early relationship in which mother and child "live and experience together." But I began to wonder, "Does this include actual physical holding?" Interestingly, Winnicott was not much more forthcoming in talking about touch in his own therapy than were the other reticent therapists I have talked about. He did not explicitly define it as part of his work in creating a holding environment. However, I did track down a case example in which he described his own use of physical as well as emotional holding:

> The detail I have chosen for description has to do with the absolute need this patient had, from time to time, to be in contact with me. Eventually it came about that she and I were together with her head in my hands. Without deliberate action on the part of either of us there developed a rocking rhythm. There we were with mutuality expressed in terms of a slight but persistent rocking movement. We were communicating without words. (quoted by Kahn in Winnicott, 1975, p. xxii)

Michael Balint, another object relations theorist, also talked about the use of touch as a part of therapy. He stated (Balint, 1968, p. 145): "The most frequent form of this contact is the holding of the analyst's hand, or one of his fingers, or touching his chair. This contact on occasion may even be highly charged, and is always vitally important for the progress of the treatment." Balint clearly pointed out the differences between this technique and that of traditional psychoanalysis: "In contrast to 'insight,' which is the result of a correct interpretation, the creation of a proper relationship results in a 'feeling'; while 'insight' correlates with seeing, 'feeling' correlates with touching" (Balint, 1968, p. 161). Object relations therapists try to facilitate new experiences as well as new thoughts. Balint was saying that touch can be a component of such a new experience.

DESCRIPTION OF THE STUDY'S SAMPLE AND METHODS

All this interested me tremendously, in terms of both the positive potential for healing and the negative potential for unclarity and even sexual abuse. I decided to research this topic by talking to women who had experienced nonerotic physical contact with their male therapists and hearing what these women themselves had to say.

"Nonerotic touch" was defined as touch that was clearly not sexual in either intent or content. Behavior such as kissing or intimate caressing was excluded from the study. But I did include touches and embraces, as long as the women felt that these had not been primarily sexual in intent.

I chose to interview women who had been in therapy with men, because I thought that it was in the dyad of female client and male therapist that Oedipal issues would be most prominent, and erotic yearnings and fears most pronounced. Each of these women had been in a therapy of at least 10 months' duration; each had terminated therapy within 2 years of the interview. They had all participated in outpatient therapy, and were all relatively well-functioning women. The study was qualitative in nature, with in-depth interviews of 10 women. Although this sample was too small to be a basis for definitive generalizations, the themes that emerged were so full of common sense and so surprisingly consistent that they merit attention as helpful guidelines for the clinician.

Six of the 10 women reported that being touched had been an unambivalently positive therapeutic experience. The other four reported mixed feelings about being touched and said that for them touch had ultimately been countertherapeutic—a definite detriment to the therapeutic relationship.

WHAT THERAPISTS DID THAT MADE TOUCH A POSITIVE OR PROBLEMATIC EXPERIENCE

As I studied the data, I began to get a sense that what made the difference between a therapeutic and a countertherapeutic experience for a client was the particular way her therapist handled the situation. There were four different kinds of therapeutic practices that seemed to affect the outcome substantially:

1. The therapist provided an environment where the client felt that she, rather than the therapist, was in control.
2. The therapist was clearly responding to the client's needs, rather than his own.
3. The therapist encouraged open discussion of the contact, rather than avoiding the topic.
4. The therapist made sure that physical and emotional intimacy developed at the same pace, rather than being insensitive to this issue of timing.

I discuss each of these in turn.

Giving the Client a Sense of Control

The six women who had experienced touch as positive and healing all felt that they had been in control of both the kind and the duration of contact. A vivid description was provided by one client, who experienced the therapist as being very sensitive to her needs in the matter of control:

> I can remember the first time that he touched me when I was very depressed. He came over to where I was sitting, and put his hands on my shoulders. And just as he was doing this, he asked me if it was all right for him to be touching me. And the respectfulness and the sensitivity with which he approached me—that in itself was very touching. He always allowed me freedom as to how much I would initiate touch, and those times when he would initiate would be times when I didn't feel connected. I would start to feel real isolated, and then he would maybe come and stand by me and touch my shoulder. And even in the touch—it was like a butterfly touch—he always left room for me to respond, to be closer or farther away, which I think is incredible.

Another woman also described being put in charge of the contact:

> He wanted me to feel in control of all of this, so I always initiated the hug. I always felt he was hugging me back. I felt that he did want me to hug him; it wasn't as if he just sort of stood there limply. But he would never prolong the hug any more than I wanted it to be, and he never cut it short. I was just real clear that I was in charge.

In contrast, none of the four women who found touch to be problematic felt in charge of the contact, or even consulted about their feelings. For each of them, touch was initiated by the therapist without asking permission and without checking whether the touching was comfortable. As an extreme example, one woman's therapist told her that touch would be beneficial. He never asked her if this were true for her or not. The point here is not that touch must always be initiated by the client, but that when it is not, the therapist must clearly communicate that the client has the right to direct the experience.

Responding to the Client's Need

The six women in the positive group felt that they had been touched solely for their own benefit. In one example, a client described the freedom of knowing that she did not have to worry about the needs of her therapist:

I never had to take care of him, or say, "Oh, my goodness, what is this going to mean? How is this going to affect him?" If I was in a place where I was clearly experiencing myself, and not really in a place to be with him, he would leave me there. When he did touch me, it didn't feel like he was requiring or requesting anything of me, or any kind of response on my part.

In sharp contrast were the reports of those who felt that physical contact had been more a need of the therapist than a response to their own needs. As noted above, one client's therapist told her that touch would be "good for her." She didn't feel that the therapist was responding only to her needs. She recalled:

He said it would help me because I was so very lonely. But I often thought that he was the lonely one.

Another client described in even more negative terms her sense that her own needs were not paramount:

I felt that I had to hug him back and be responsive to his physical gestures of affection. Because I did feel like a lot of it came out of unexamined needs of his own—that he was someone that wanted a lot of warmth and love and affection in his life. I mean, I never got out of my chair and went to hug him. I didn't say to him, "I feel like I wish you'd hug me." I mean, whose need was that? It wasn't my need; it was his need. It was his need. I don't know—that makes me very angry.

Encouraging Open Discussion of Touch

The six women in the positive group had all discussed the experience of touch with their therapists. Their discussions included both a clarification of the boundaries and limits of the relationship, and an exploration of the possible sexual feelings that might be aroused. Here is how one client, who had an extremely positive therapeutic outcome, described her initial anxiety regarding touch. After several sessions in which the therapist had held her when she was very upset, he raised the issue of touch and sexuality:

He gave me permission to have these feelings, and [said] that it was sort of like a normal thing that would come up if you're working really deeply. Those feelings are going to surface. And [he also said] that I wasn't a bad person because I was feeling sexual.

In this case, the therapist was also able to discuss the limits and boundaries of their relationship in away that made her feel safe.

A second positive report came from a woman who had ample reason to be afraid and vigilant, having just come from a therapy with a seductive male therapist. She found great comfort in her new therapist's constantly checking with her about the meaning of their contact. She said:

> I knew that he did care about me a lot, but it was very clear that the love and caring was therapeutic. I think the more we talked about that, the better I felt. And he would always ask. When he would put his hands on my shoulders, he would say, "Is this raising anxiety?" He even said things like, when he was moving away, you know, he wanted to know how I was feeling. He clearly didn't want me to feel that I was being left or that kind of thing.

In marked contrast to these experiences, the four women who found touch to be countertherapeutic never had such discussions with their therapists. Thus, the limits of these relationships were never discussed; the clients never had a chance to explore their own feelings. This left them feeling unsafe. One client described her uneasiness and confusion this way:

> I didn't feel that this [holding her and stroking her hair] was just as far as he would go. I had no idea how far he would go. And it left me really frightened at his lack of definition of boundaries. It felt dangerous to me, although nothing [sexual] had ever really happened.

Another client angrily described how her therapist never asked her how she felt about the hugs that he would sometimes initiate in their sessions, and that he always gave her at the end of each interview:

> I find it kind of incredible when I think back that he didn't even ever ask me what that meant to me, how I felt about having him touch me—that it was just done with some implicit assumption that we knew each other well enough now, that that was OK, and that it was an expression of affection. I mean, he never even checked out what it meant to me.

Keeping Physical and Emotional Intimacy Congruent

The six women in the positive group felt that physical intimacy proceeded at about the same pace as the emotional intimacy. The therapists were sensitive to the degree of trust and intimacy the relationships had achieved, and were also sensitive about the relation of touch to the issues being worked through at the time. Here is how one client described this parallel growth of physical and emotional contact, which was essential to her ability to trust:

> In the beginning, there wasn't a lot of contact. But as our relationship grew, the quality of our touching changed. In the fourth year, we'd come to a kind of understanding about what the boundaries were and what was OK. I remember having a very deep experience, and he just stood up and gave me a real strong embrace, which felt very good. But if he'd done that even a year before, it would have felt very intrusive. Too much for me. I would have been frightened about the sexuality of it. But given our relationship and my own sense of my own boundaries, and his clarity, it clearly was a very human, caring contact. So somehow the touching grew congruently as our relationship grew. There was no inconsistency about the way he touched me and the way our relationship was emerging. That seemed important.

Another woman, whose experience was also positive, was aware of her therapist's sensitivity to timing in a slightly different way. He had noticed immediately that she was uncomfortable when he put his hand on hers in a comforting gesture. It was he who raised the issue, and by doing so, allowed her to tell him that the touch was painful. As she reported it:

> It felt like saying, here was affection, but when the hand was withdrawn it was like the affection was taken away.

The therapist didn't use touch again until the client herself requested it a year later. She said that she needed to work through her feeling of extreme isolation and vulnerability before she could benefit from the comfort of physical contact. As she gradually emerged from her strongly defended shell, she needed physical warmth and could tolerate it.

For the four women with problematic experiences, no mention was made of the touch being geared sensitively to their needs in this area of timing.

THE POSITIVE FUNCTIONS OF TOUCH

So far, I've discussed how touch can be used in a sensitive way that is helpful to the client (i.e., what the therapist can do). Now I'd like to talk more specifically about the functions that touch had for the six women in the positive group—those who felt that touch made a significant contribution to their therapeutic experiences. In listening to the responses of these six clients, I found three important categories of positive meaning:

1. Touch prevented a client from becoming lost in her pain by providing a link to external reality.
2. Touch communicated acceptance, resulting in greater self-esteem.
3. Touch allowed a client to experience new modes of relating.

Here is an elaboration of each of these points.

Providing a Link to External Reality

Four of the six positive respondents said that touch provided a connection to external reality when they felt chaotic inside. The physical contact helped them to keep from getting lost in pain that was at times excruciating. In a striking example, one client described how touch was sometimes necessary to keep her from becoming overwhelmed by strong emotions. She said of her therapist:

> He taught me that I didn't have to get isolated in this awful pain at the exclusion of this person who was really caring about me. His physical contact reminded me he was really there. And that was significant, and it was also a way when even in between sessions, if I had a hard time, the memory of that physical touch would help me remember that he existed in the world too. The physical contact would just be a graphic way of remembering that I could be in contact with external reality, something outside of myself and my feelings.

Several women in this group emphasized that touch created the actual experience of not being isolated at a time when words alone would have seemed like meaningless reassurance. They were referring to deep experiences in which language, a more adult form of communication, would not have been adequate. Because touch is a more direct way of speaking to the younger or more fragmented self that sometimes emerges as a part of treatment, it can express a sense of relatedness that words alone may not adequately convey.

Communicating Acceptance and Increasing Self-Esteem

Of the six positive respondents, five said that they felt an increase of self-esteem as a result of their physical contact. One example was provided by a woman who entered therapy feeling unloved and unlovable, and found that physical contact with her therapist spoke directly to this issue. She said:

> The issue was my self-worth, and whether I was lovable. And that's what the pain was all about, and that's what the physical comforting addressed. At some point I began to feel that I was a worthy person—that I must deserve that love that I was getting from him.

Interestingly, it wasn't just the women in the positive group who felt that touch had enhanced their self-esteem. All of the women in the problematic group also felt increased self-esteem and confidence as one result of the warmth and touching in their therapies. In those cases, unfortunately, the enhanced self-esteem was counterbalanced by other difficulties in the therapeutic relationship. I will explain the dynamics of this process shortly.

Allowing the Experience of New Modes of Relating

The third and last function of touch was that it allowed clients to experience new modes of relating. Let me discuss what these new modes were.

1. One woman was able, for the first time, to experience a person in authority as giving rather than demanding affection. This example is particularly interesting because—unlike the other nine clients, for whom touch was used repeatedly in the course of therapy—this woman was the only client for whom touch was used just once. Her experience testifies to the power of even a single experience of touch. This particular client had experienced her parents as controlling and demanding. When her therapist resisted her wish to end therapy, she began to see him in the same way. He felt that termination was premature, and began to struggle with her and demand that she stay. Fortunately, he figured out what was going on and was able to change his behavior. He let her terminate without struggling with her. What she remembered most vividly about this changed interaction was the therapist's spontaneous embrace at the last session. She felt that this act communicated, even more clearly than their discussions, that he was willing to give to her without first having to receive. She was grateful for that embrace and the message she felt it contained.

2. Two women learned to reach out rather than withdraw when they were experiencing pain. One of these women had the experience of being "coached" by her therapist. He taught her to ask for the

specific form of physical comforting she wanted, such as sitting beside him with her head on his shoulder and being held. She said:

> These experiences of reaching out and being able to get physical warmth have been the first times when I've actively turned to somebody and said "Help me," instead of withdrawing and curling up in a ball and putting up signs saying "Leave me alone."

3. Two other women learned that they could have relationships that included both closeness and respect for the separate needs of each individual. Touch intensified and condensed this experience of having intimacy and yet at the same time experiencing differentiation.

4. Finally, one woman emphasized that her physical relationship with her therapist was her first experience that physical contact and sexuality are not necessarily the same thing. She came from a strict, repressive home, where she had learned that all touch was dangerously sexual. She had felt confused and hurt and somehow guilty when her father had turned away from her during her adolescence. Her new experience with the therapist was a revelation that she could be close to a man who did not view her as a dangerously sexual being. She said:

> The physical contact was an essential part of my learning about relationships—The whole thing of various kinds of touch and various qualities of touch and various degrees of intimacy. That never got differentiated in my own mind until I was in this relationship with my therapist. I knew intellectually, but I didn't experience until then what it was like to be close to someone and not necessarily have to be sexual at all.

We've seen how the positive experience of touch enriched the therapies for these six women and added a dimension not available through words alone. Now I'd like to turn to the last portion of my data and discuss more fully the experiences of those who felt that touch was mainly countertherapeutic.

THE MEANING OF TOUCH FOR THOSE WHO EXPERIENCED TOUCH AS COUNTERTHERAPEUTIC

Each of the four participants in this study who experienced touch as mainly countertherapeutic did feel that some aspects of their therapies were worthwhile. Yet they shared a strong ambivalence about touch and related issues. Significantly, not one of them was able to talk to her therapist about this ambivalence. This fact underlines the power of the therapy experience: All of these women were bright and articulate, yet none of them felt able to confront the issue of the unwelcome touching. Four themes emerged that help explain the meaning of the touching for these women and that shed light on the reasons for their silence:

1. Being touched made the clients feel loved and worthwhile; consequently, they were reluctant to bring up negative feelings or concerns that might jeopardize these feelings.
2. Each woman felt angry at her therapist, but guilty about the anger and reluctant to express it.
3. The therapists were perceived as needy and vulnerable, and hence as in need of protection from the clients' negative feelings.
4. The therapy in each case tended to recapitulate the dynamics of the woman's family of origin, rather than to help resolve them.

What follows is an elaboration of each of these themes.

Reluctance to Jeopardize Positive Feelings

All four women for whom touch had been primarily countertherapeutic felt that the emotional and physical warmth of their therapists had made them feel special and loved, and these feelings in turn contributed to a feeling of greater self-worth. There was, however, a catch: This warmth was so gratifying that it became impossible to bring up negative feelings or concerns. One woman explained:

> What began to happen was that I came to look for it, to expect it, and to want it. I didn't want to want it. But it had a momentum of its own. I wanted to be unique, to be most special to him, to make him into the caring father I never had. I felt that it was weird—that what we were doing was wrong—but I didn't want it to stop.

Anger, and Guilt about Anger

The anger these women felt stemmed from the fact that they didn't feel free to bring up negative or ambivalent feelings, and from the failure of the therapists to ask what the touch meant to the clients. The women were also resentful because they realized that there was an unclarity about boundaries and sexual limits, and that this was harmful to the therapeutic work. Yet several women felt guilty about this resentment because they perceived the therapists as kind and giving. One client described her dilemma like this:

> He was so loving and so caring that I felt incredibly guilty for having the negative feelings. I really felt that the negative, bad feelings were just not allowed because this person was so—cared for me so much. How could I be such a horrible person as to have these negative feelings?

Another woman said that her guilt at feeling angry stemmed not so much from her feeling that the therapist was kind and giving, but from her assumption that she must be the one who was wrong. Her low self-esteem and her acceptance of authority combined to make her discount her sense that the therapist was acting inappropriately. She therefore felt guilty at the resentment that began gradually to emerge.

Perception of Therapists as Needy and Vulnerable

These women found themselves unable to confront their therapists because the therapists were perceived as needy and vulnerable. This was a role reversal in which the clients found themselves in the role of caretakers. One woman linked this reversal directly to the touching that had occurred. She felt that the relationship between her and the therapist became more mutual as a result of the physical contact, and that consequently the traditional roles became less clear.

Another respondent said that the greater intimacy that came about from the physical contact was very gratifying. She felt eager to be close to this man for whom she cared so deeply. Later he began to share some of his own problems with her. Even though she realized that this role reversal was inappropriate, she wanted to provide support for him. As a result, she lost the therapeutic relationship: This man could no longer be an objectively loving presence who had only her best interests at heart.

All four of these women felt that their therapists had been initially available to them, and had been primarily concerned about their needs. Over time, however, each client shifted toward more of a caretaking role. In each case, touch helped create both the intimacy and the confusion that resulted in the reversal of roles.

Recapitulation of Family-of-Origin Dynamics

Not surprisingly, a fourth factor that maintained the relationship despite ambivalence in each of these cases was that the therapy in some way recapitulated the dynamics in the woman's family of origin. For example, one woman had been the oldest child in her family, and so had taken on the role of caretaker and peacemaker. In her therapy, she took up this role again, but was unable to work it through because of her therapist's needs. For another woman, the central dynamic was her inability to separate adequately from a fused relationship with her mother. Just as she had difficulty in leaving home, she had a hard time separating from the therapeutic relationship because of the yearnings aroused in her by its deep intimacy.

Two other women were working on unresolved relationships with fathers who had been at once warm and intrusive. One especially remembered the satisfaction of being her father's favorite. She also remembered the intrusive, inappropriately exciting, and frightening quality of his touch. She felt that her therapist was trying to provide her with a corrective emotional experience. That is, he was trying to show that touch could be both warm and gentle, and that she need no longer fear being physically close. However, he created a situation, in the client's words, that was "really just the same."

In each of these therapies—in which touch was experienced as ultimately countertherapeutic—there was great ambivalence. Touch served to heighten a sense of shared warmth and personal acceptance, but was experienced much more strongly as confusing, intrusive, and anxiety-provoking. In none of these therapies did the client raise the subject of her discomfort, for the reasons just discussed. And the therapists in these cases never asked whether there were negative facets of these experiences.

SUMMARY AND CONCLUSIONS

In summary, this study shows that touch has the power to create both therapeutic and countertherapeutic outcomes. It is clear that to be of therapeutic value, touch must be used with great care. It is equally clear that to condemn touch without exception is to rob psychotherapy of a powerful tool for healing. I'd like to underscore those findings that can serve the clinician as guidelines for the use of touch.

First, the client should be in control of the experience. From time to time, many therapists find it useful to take control, pushing or confronting clients about certain issues. Touch, however, should not be forced. It needs to be consonant with a client's needs for and ability to accept this form of intimacy.

Second, touch should not be experienced as a need or demand of the therapist. Of course, a therapist should always take care to separate his or her own needs from those of the client. But in the case of touch—which is so highly laden with emotional meanings—it is even more essential for the therapist to be clear.

Third, physical contact must be discussed. This is crucially important. The limits and boundaries of the experience, as well as its possible sexual aspects, must be explored. This discussion should not be confined to a single exploration of the issue. Ongoing discussion should occur, especially when either the client or the therapist changes his or her behavior—whether this means more, less, or a different kind of touching.

Fourth, good timing is essential. It was important to the women who had positive experiences that physical and emotional intimacy proceeded congruently. Similarly, some women reported that it was important that their therapists were sensitive to the relationships between touch and the issues being discussed in the work. This means that the clinician needs to be attuned to the development of the therapeutic relationship as experienced by the client, as well as sensitive to the issues that are salient in the therapy at the time.

In addition to—and, it may seem, in spite of—the above-described considerations, touch should be part of a spontaneous and genuine interaction. It should emerge not from a theoretical position, but from an immediate need of the client and a genuine response of the therapist. Yet, like all other aspects of therapy, it needs to be embedded in the context of a careful assessment of the client's needs and reactions. In other words, it is part of our complex, difficult, and rewarding mission as therapists of fully using both our hearts and our heads.

ACKNOWLEDGMENT

This chapter is based on my doctoral dissertation, submitted in partial fulfillment of the requirements for the EdD degree at Boston University, 1981.

REFERENCES

Balint, M. (1968). *The basic fault: Therapeutic aspects of regression.* London: Tavistock.

Forer, B. (1969). The taboo against touching in psychotherapy. *Psychotherapy: Theory, Research, and Practice, 6*(4), 229–231.

Jones, E. (1955). *The life and work of Sigmund Freud: Vol. 2. Years of maturity.* New York: Basic Books.

Jordan, M. (1970). Supervision of a defensive non-verbal communication. *Voices,* 5(36), 7–13.

Menninger, K. (1958). *Theory of psychoanalytic technique.* New York: Basic Books.

Older, J. (1977). Four taboos that may limit the success of psychotherapy. *Psychiatry, 40,* 197–203.

Tyson, C. (1979). Physical contact in psychotherapy. *Dissertation Abstracts International, 39*(9-B), 4601.

Winnicott, D. W. (1958). The theory of parent–infant relationship. *International Journal of Psycho-Analysis, 41,* 585–595.

Winnicott, D. W. (1975). *Through pediatrics to psychoanalysis.* New York: Basic Books.

Wolberg, L. R. (1954). *The technique of psychotherapy.* New York: Grune & Stratton.

FURTHER RESEARCH ON THE PATIENT'S EXPERIENCE OF TOUCH IN PSYCHOTHERAPY

Judith Horton

Little attention has been given to actual patients' experiences of touch in individual psychotherapy, other than to reports of the sequelae of sexual intimacy between therapist and patient. Yet research indicates that the patient's point of view is a valuable source of information in assessing therapeutic alliance (TA) and predicting therapy outcome (Gurman, 1977; Hartley & Strupp, 1983; Marziali, 1984; Salvio, Beutler, Wood, & Engle, 1992). Furthermore, much of the research on touch in therapy has consisted of analogue studies that artificially apply a touch "condition" to pseudopatients or short-term counseling volunteers (Alagna, Whitcher, Fisher, & Wicas, 1979; Hubble, Noble, & Robinson, 1981; Pattison, 1973; Stockwell & Dye, 1980; Tyson, 1978). These studies fail to capture the dynamic meaning of touch in real therapeutic encounters; their generalizability to ongoing psychotherapy in which touch is sensitively timed and integral to the patient's needs and issues is therefore questionable.

Geib's (1982) phenomenological study of patients' evaluation and meanings attributed to physical contact occurring in ongoing therapy is perhaps the best source of empirical data we have regarding the impact of touch in therapy. A limitation of her study is its small, homogeneous sample—10 relatively young, white, female patients of

male, traditional therapists (psychodynamically oriented "talk" therapists not explicitly offering touch as a therapeutic technique). Geib
found five factors associated with patients' positive or negative evaluations of touch in therapy, and identified a number of themes associated with the positive or negative valence of touch.

My study questioned whether four of Geib's factors would be
reflected in a larger, more diverse sample of patients and therapists.
(The fifth factor—whether the patient's expectations of therapy or the
therapist were fulfilled by the reality of the therapist—was not included
because it was considered too difficult to define in questionnaire
format. It is also not discussed in Chapter 8). The factors examined
were: (1) clarity of communication regarding touch, sexual feelings, and
boundaries of therapy (including the patient's sense that the boundaries, when not explicitly discussed, were clear and unambiguous); (2)
the patient's perception of control in initiating and sustaining physical
contact; (3) congruence of touch with the level of intimacy in the
relationship and with the patient's particular issues; and (4) the patient's perception that the physical contact was for his or her benefit,
rather than the therapist's.

In addition, I wanted to look at another, more general area of
potential relevance in understanding patients' responses to touch in
therapy—level of TA. Bordin (1976) identified three components of TA:
the agreement between therapist and patient about (1) the goals and
(2) the tasks of therapy, which he believed mediated the quality of (3)
the relationship or bond. TA has only recently been defined empirically
and tested (Alexander & Luborsky, 1986; Horvath & Greenberg, 1986,
1989; Luborsky, Crits-Christoph, Alexander, Margolis, & Cohen, 1983;
Marmor, Horowitz, Weiss, & Marziali, 1986; Marziali, 1984). TA measures have been shown to predict treatment outcome measures, with
the patient's perspective being especially valuable in predicting outcome (Bachelor, 1991).

Logically, degree of TA should be predictive of patients' evaluations of physical contact in therapy, since TA is indicative of the
quality of the bond between patient and therapist, as well as of general
agreement on the tasks of therapy (which might include the use of
touch). I used the patient portion of the Working Alliance Inventory
(WAI) developed by Horvath and Greenberg (1986) as my measure of
TA, because it is relatively brief, can be self-administered, is divided
into subscales corresponding to the conceptual components of TA
suggested by Bordin (1976), and has been shown to be significantly
correlated with outcome in therapy (Horvath & Greenberg, 1989).

A third area I wanted to assess was whether greater potential for
sexual attraction in the therapy dyad—for instance, when a heterosexual

patient is paired with an opposite-sex therapist—makes touch more ambiguous and prone to misinterpretation, and thus less likely to be positively evaluated. A study of nonverbal communication (Heslin & Alper, 1983) found that females' generally positive reactions to being touched were less favorable when the toucher was a male other than their partner. It seems logical to conclude that discomfort with touch in therapy may be more likely when there is an increased potential for sexual attraction.

METHODS AND PROCEDURES

An anonymous survey seemed the least intrusive way to reach a large, heterogeneous sample of actual psychotherapy patients. In order to reach a diverse cross-section of patients (and therapists), I gathered a list of therapists in a large Southern metropolitan area from state professional association and telephone directories of therapists working with adults. Over 300 therapists were contacted, and 900 research packets were distributed. To maximize chances of getting negative as well as positive evaluations of therapist touch, I attempted to reach some patients other than through their therapists. I distributed research packets through a network of free support groups for sexual abuse survivors and in a variety of nontherapy settings, such as churches, bookstores, Twelve-Step groups, and support groups. I also advertised for patient volunteers in several weekly newspapers.

The research packet consisted of a cover letter explaining the purpose of the study, a 36-item questionnaire that I developed, and a TA measure (the client portion of the WAI). A postage-paid, self-addressed envelope was included so that patients could mail the packet directly to me. Volunteers were reassured of the voluntary and confidential nature of their participation in the study, and were instructed *not* to put their names or those of their therapists on any of the materials.

The study targeted patients who had had a *significant* positive or negative experience of touch in therapy, or for whom touch was a salient issue. The cover letter and questionnaire both stated the criteria for participation in the study: Participation was restricted to adults (20 years or older) who were or had been within the last 2 years in individual therapy with a non-body-oriented psychotherapist for at least 2 months and had experienced some sort of physical contact with this therapist (beyond accidental contact or a formal handshake). Only those who returned *both* the questionnaire (specifically evaluating the valence of touch in therapy) and the WAI were included in the study.

The questionnaire gathered patient demographics and asked about the main issues or problems patients were working on in therapy. Each patient's attitudes toward and receptivity to physical contact with the therapist were then assessed by asking the following questions:

Have you ever wanted your therapist to hug, hold, or touch you in some way?
Have you ever asked (directly or indirectly) for physical contact with your therapist?
If so, were you comfortable with your therapist's response?

Patients were then asked to evaluate on a 7-point Likert scale (from "very negative" to "very positive") their overall response to the physical contact that occurred in their therapy, and whether their feelings about themselves, about their therapists, or about the quality of therapeutic work were positively affected by the touch. Other Likert items assessed the factors Geib (1982) identified as associated with patients' evaluations of touch occurring in therapy. Touch in previous therapy, if it had occurred, was also evaluated. A number of therapist variables were gathered as well. Finally, short-answer, open-ended questions allowed patients to illustrate or elaborate on their answers to scaled items.

RESULTS OF THE STUDY

Of the 231 completed research packets returned, the majority were from patients who were in therapy with private practitioners (94%), most often with doctoral-level psychologists (56%). The respondents were predominantly white (90%), generally in their 30s or 40s, and well educated. Significantly more females (84%) than males (16%) responded; the majority of female patients saw female therapists (84%), and the majority of males saw male therapists (68%). All combinations of patient sexual orientation and gender with therapist gender were reported, except for a bisexual male or female seeing an opposite-sex therapist.

The problems most often listed as presenting problems or main issues of therapy were relational difficulties (48%); sexual abuse (incest, childhood sexual abuse, unspecified sexual abuse, or rape) was the second largest category, with a third of the participants reporting such issues. There were an additional 64 references to trauma-based problems or diagnoses, including physical and emotional abuse or neglect, posttraumatic stress disorder, and multiple personality disorder. Depression, grief, or loss (29%) ranked third. Self issues, such as low self-esteem, shame, "false self," and learning to assert oneself, represented the next largest group of complaints at 28%. (These figures represent the percentages of total surveys returned that listed these symptoms or presenting problems. Patients were not limited to listing only one symptom; therefore, percentages do not equal 100%.)

An additional source of information regarding the symptoms or issues prompting therapy was a symptom checklist. Respondents who left the question about presenting problems blank checked several problems here. The checklist indicated a considerably higher prevalence of depression, self-esteem issues, isolation or loneliness, and anxiety than was indicated in responses to the question regarding presenting problems.

The results confirmed that three of Geib's (1982) four factors were significantly correlated with patients' positive evaluations of touch occurring in therapy. A stepwise multiple-regression procedure yielded three predictive or explanatory variables, which entered in the following order: (1) congruence of touch with the patient's issues; (2) the patient's perception of the therapist's sensitivity to his or her reaction to touch; and (3) the patient's ability to communicate with the therapist about feelings toward the therapist. Together, these three variables accounted for 29% of the variance in the overall evaluation of touch occurring in therapy. Whether the patient felt the touch was for his or her benefit was the only one of Geib's factors that did not attain significance.

Other potentially significant factors, such as patient or therapist gender, patient sexual orientation or age, and patient–therapist age difference, were not shown to affect patient evaluation of touch. An additional stepwise regression analysis showed that patient endorsement of wanting therapist touch (which is, in a sense, a measure of its congruence) and congruence with level of intimacy in the relationship improved predictive ability from 29% to 44%.

A series of t tests on all variables considered also found that none of the above-mentioned factors (age, gender, gender combination in dyad, etc.) were associated with a significantly more positive evaluation of touch. Three groups of problems endorsed on the problem checklist, however, were found to be related to a significantly more positive evaluation of touch: sexual problems; history of sexual abuse; and fears/phobias. (Anxiety and a history of physical abuse/neglect came very close to meeting the .05 level.) Unfortunately, the narrative data did not clarify why those reporting fears/phobias and sexual problems rated therapist touch more positively than did those not reporting these symptoms. The narrative answers did shed light on the more positive evaluation of touch by sexual abuse survivors.

The reparative effect of touch for some patients was strongly indicated by the narrative responses of patients reporting childhood sexual and/or physical abuse. Of the patients who reported a history of abuse (sexual abuse, n = 43; physical abuse and/or neglect, n = 30; both sexual and physical abuse, n = 50), 71% (87 respondents) wrote that touch repaired self-esteem, trust, and a sense of their own power or agency, especially in setting limits and asking for what they needed. Many described learning through touch in therapy that nurturing need not be sexual, and that they were deserving of nurturing.

The qualitative information gathered from patients' answers to open-ended questions was thematized, tabulated, and compared with the positive and negative themes identified by Geib (1982). If the narrative description did not contain key words or phrases, and its meaning was not clear, it was ignored and not counted.

A very large number of written descriptions pointed to two important themes. The first of these themes—that touch created a feeling of bond, closeness, or a sense that the therapist really cared, thereby facilitating increased trust and openness—was reported by 69% of the sample (n = 159). This theme was expressed in these ways: "made therapy feel personal rather than business-like"; "made me feel cared for . . . felt very connected to my therapist"; "assured me of her presence during the session, and her commitment to go through the process of healing with me." The second theme—that touch communicated acceptance and enhanced the patient's self-esteem—was reported by 47% of the sample (n = 109). This theme was expressed in words such as these: "made me feel safe with her, important and precious to her"; "helped me learn that I was lovable"; "means validation and unconditional care." This theme was also identified in Geib's (1982) study.

Multiple themes were identified in the narrative descriptions, so these two major themes cannot be looked at additively. Rather, they seemed to form the core of a cluster of themes having to do with the quality of the bond in therapy (a sense that the therapist was emotionally involved and reliable), and with the perceived benefit to the patient of enhanced self-esteem, trust, and ability to "open up" and use therapy more profitably.

Respectful, reassuring touch seemed to help many patients feel supported and safe enough to move into threatening material or a deeper level. One woman wrote that "by making me feel safe and loved, [touch] allowed me to move forward at times when I didn't think the pain would allow it. . . . It has been one of the most healing parts of my therapy." Another described how her therapist "would hold me as I cried, mourned, wailed during sessions, and would give strong hugs at the end of each session. I could not have done the life-changing work I did were it not for the physical support of that therapist." A number of patients expressed their belief that touch was a more reliable gauge than words. One patient wrote, "The mouth can lie, but the body can't." Another noted that she "trusted her [therapist's] touch long before I could trust or even really listen to her words."

Only 10 respondents gave descriptions of negative experiences of touch in current therapy. Four females and two males described therapist behavior that signaled to them their current therapists' discomfort with touch (only one indicated that this was eventually discussed and was no longer confusing). Three females and one male indicated that touch (or the kind of touch) was accepted or tolerated, but was not offered to meet an expressed need of theirs. Other references to discomfort with touch in the current therapy were qualified by descriptions of how this had been beneficially resolved, or by notes that the discomfort was an issue these patients sought to work through in therapy.

References to unwelcome, intrusive, seductive, or outright sexualized touch from previous therapists were made by 13% of the sample. These experiences were rated from "negative" to "very negative," and were generally described as either "confusing" or "very destructive." Several patients discussed their previous therapists' assuming a level of intimacy and familiarity with touch that, though not sexual in nature, was nonetheless offensive and caused them to flee therapy.

A high degree of TA (as indicated by WAI score) was also shown to be positively related to positive evaluation of touch in therapy ($r = .32$, $p = .0001$). When the WAI's three subscales were considered, Bond was the one significant variable accounting for the patient's positive evaluation of touch.

Results did not support the negative effect of hypothesized increased potential for sexual attraction on the patient's evaluation of touch. A t test comparing groups—"high potential for attraction," defined as patient paired with "object choice" (i.e., heterosexual patient with opposite-sex therapist or homosexual patient with same-sex therapist), and "low potential for attraction," defined as the inverse—found no significant difference between groups.

An optional, specific question about how openly sexual feelings between therapist and patient were addressed was answered by fewer than 28% of the respondents, too few to allow for its inclusion in the analysis. Surprisingly, even patients who answered the question the most negatively ("not at all openly"), nonetheless rated their overall response to touch in therapy positively. Of the 14 patients who reported that sexual feelings were not addressed openly in their current therapy, none rated therapist touch negatively, and only 1 rated it as neither positive nor negative.

DISCUSSION

Although the results support Geib's (1982) findings that patients' positive evaluations of touch in therapy are associated with its congruence, the patient's sense of control, and the patient's ability to speak freely with the therapist, the narrative answers indicate that many patients have difficulty both verbally requesting physical contact and expressing negative reactions about the therapy. In this light, it seems especially important that touch be neither gratuitous nor exploitative, but a genuine response to the patient's expressed or manifest need for physical contact.

A perception of their therapists' sensitivity to their reaction to touch seems to bolster many patients' sense of control by reassuring them that their nonverbal message has been "heard" and respected. Sensitivity to subtle nonverbal messages may preclude incongruent touch, in that a therapist senses when touch is unwelcome, or, when eliciting an ambivalent or negative response to touch, desists and explores the reaction.

In general, touch is likely to be perceived positively when there is sufficient intimacy in the therapy relationship to enable the patient to communicate on a deeper level about the therapy relationship. Openness is a hallmark of intimacy. Yet the ability to communicate intimate thoughts and feelings *about the therapist to the therapist* is not something one can readily expect from many patients. It is often the product of a well-established, successful therapy, or of skillful facilitation by the therapist. Ironically, touch itself may play an important role in facilitating such openness. More than two-thirds of the respondents wrote that touch communicated or reinforced a sense that their therapists genuinely cared, and that the safety created by this bond helped them open up, go deeper, and take risks.

Interestingly, Geib (1982) noted that the inverse of openness—a patient's *inability* to speak openly with a therapist about the therapy relationship—was involved in negative experiences and evaluations of touch. Without facilitation by the therapist, or a level of intimacy in which the patient feels free to communicate potentially uncomfortable, embarrassing, or negative thoughts and feelings about the therapy or therapist, physical contact is apt to be risky; in such a situation, how can fears, concerns, and negative reactions be addressed? Geib (1982) grouped the negative responses to therapist touch she found in her study under the general umbrella of "ambivalence and silence." Often touch had been appreciated or helpful, but inability to address concerns about touch eventually led to a negative appraisal of its effect.

A patient's perception that touch was for the patient's, not the therapist's benefit was the only one of Geib's variables that was not found to be significant in accounting for the patients' positive evaluation of touch in our study. Geib found the inverse of this factor to be associated with negative reactions to therapist touch. The fact that there were very few negative evaluations of current therapist touch in the present study may explain why it did not enter the equation as a highly significant variable. Patients may be more likely to evaluate touch negatively when they feel that touch *primarily* meets the needs of their therapists, but may evaluate it neutrally or positively in the absence of this impression.

The majority of patients indicated in their narrative answers that touch helped them feel a bond with their therapists. Descriptions of the therapy relationship that were used to express this concept included "bond," "safety," "closeness," "there for me," "on my side," "deepened trust," "really cares about me," and "able to handle strong feelings." For many, touch directly communicated, through their therapists' willingness, sincerity, or lack of hesitation, the therapists' acceptance or positive regard for them, despite their own self-doubts and self-loathing. Feeling "touchable" allowed some patients to feel better about themselves by offering a sense of parity with their therapists, and lessening self-consciousness and shame in revealing hidden or denied aspects of self.

It is not surprising that a high WAI score was positively related to positive evaluation of touch in therapy, or that the Bond subscale was the most significant. Both theoretical literature and studies measuring TA and therapeutic outcome stress the centrality of the therapist–patient bond. Bachelor's (1991) study of the relationship between patient improvement (specific measures of therapeutic outcome) and three different measures of TA found that patient perception of the therapist and the degree of bond "yielded the stronger predictions and involved therapist-offered helpfulness, warmth and emotional involvement, and exploratory interventions" (p. 534). She concluded that "the therapeutically most relevant factors are therapist-provided help and demonstrated warmth, caring, and emotional involvement," which "appear to enhance the client's collaboration and commitment to the process" (p. 546).

The majority of themes identified in the narrative responses had to do with the quality of the bond in therapy—a patient's sense that a therapist was emotionally involved and reliable, and the perceived benefit of enhanced self-esteem, trust, and increased ability to "open up" and use therapy more profitably. These findings seem to confirm Bachelor's (1991) assessment of the importance of therapeutic alliance from the patient's perspective, especially the bond fostered by the perception of therapist warmth, involvement, and positive regard. Damaging themes most often mentioned in reference to previous therapies were either examples of empathic failures, or actual violations of a patient's trust. Clearly, sexualized touch in therapy, like a rotten apple in a barrel of apples, spoils the good.

It is noteworthy that the problems or issues most frequently reported by respondents as presenting problems or issues being addressed in therapy were those for which interpersonal touch has been theoretically cited as potentially beneficial: intimacy and relational difficulties, abuse, isolation or loneliness, depression or grief, and self-esteem and identity issues (Hollender, 1970; Hollender & Mercer, 1976; Lowen, 1967; Mintz, 1969; Robertiello, 1974a, 1974b; Shepherd, 1979; Stein & Sanfilippo, 1985; Wilson, 1982).

An important and unexpected finding of this study was the significantly more positive evaluation of touch in therapy by those reporting abuse, sexual or otherwise. Their narrative answers clarified that respectful touch directly communicated, in ways that verbal reassurances at times could not, two critical messages. First, it communicated that they were "lovable," as one woman put it—"worthy of a clean, pure touch" that did not carry "the high cost of losing myself." A mundane but profound revelation for many abuse survivors was that they deserved to be nurtured. Second, respectful touch had the ability, as one respondent stated, to communicate or teach "on an integrated level ... appropriate boundaries." In terms of trust or belief, experiencing was believing for these respondents.

QUESTIONS RAISED BY THE STUDY

Although a large number of research packets were distributed to a variety of therapy settings and support groups, and through newspaper solicitation of volunteers, very few of the questionnaires returned contained descriptions of negative touch or unfavorable evaluations of touch in *current* therapy. This is perhaps the most serious limitation of the present study. Almost two-thirds of the sample ($n = 156$) gave the highest possible score to the question "How would you characterize your overall response to the touching that has occurred in your therapy?" The results therefore speak only to positive evaluations of touch in therapy; no generalizations can be made about negative evaluations of touch, other than to point to common themes mentioned by patients describing their current or previous therapy. Other than Geib's (1982) limited sample, there is no systematic documentation from the patient's perspective of negative touch experiences in therapy.

Unfortunately, there are no statistics available to permit me to determine how representative this sample was of the larger outpatient therapy population. Although overall there was considerable diversity in sample characteristics, certain comparisons could not be made because the sample was predominantly white and female. Questions remain regarding possible gender and ethnic (or cultural) differences in receptivity to touch in therapy.

Is the high percentage of women represented here an artifact of sampling, or does it point to actual gender differences in touch in psychotherapy? One reason more females than males may have responded to this survey is that several low-cost women's clinics and a network of sexual abuse survivors' groups (which are predominantly female) distributed packets, whereas no comparable agencies treating males were identified. Surveys of therapists' attitudes and behaviors (Holroyd & Brodsky, 1977; Milakovich, 1992), however, indicate that female therapists report engaging in more nurturant touch than male therapists, and more often with same-sex than with opposite-sex patients. Male therapists were noted in Holroyd and Brodsky's (1977) survey to be more likely to perceive benefit in nonerotic touching of opposite-sex patients, but also to perceive a greater risk of misunderstanding of nonerotic touch by patients of either sex.

Women are probably more frequently touched in therapy than men, and more frequently by female than by male therapists; however, incidence of touch was not accessed in this study, and further research is needed to support a conclusion that women receive more nurturing touch in therapy than men do. Men and women are socialized differently, especially with regard to expressive, receptive, and sexual behavior (Abbey & Melby, 1986; Nguyen, Heslin, & Nguyen, 1975). Despite the fact that no significant gender differences were found in this study, potential gender differences in desire for and response to touch in therapy warrant further investigation.

The finding that sexual orientation and gender pairing in the therapy dyad did not affect a patient's evaluation of touch in therapy is interesting; yet, in retrospect, these factors probably did not adequately tap the sexual tension and ambiguity of intent they were intended to tap. Many other factors bear on the issue of sexual tension in the therapy relationship: whether or not the therapist or the patient is *actually* attracted and consciously or unconsciously signaling interest;

whether the patient feels threatened by this attraction; the overlapping relevance of other factors studied, such as the therapist's clarity of communication regarding boundaries and the patient's ability to be self-revealing about potentially awkward or embarrassing sexual feelings and thoughts; and the potential for primitive longings for merger with the therapist, regardless of gender or sexual orientation, to be confused with adult sexual feelings.

It appears that neither *potential for sexual feelings* in therapy (as indicated by gender and sexual orientation pairing of therapists and patients), nor *actual unacknowledged sexual feelings* (reported by patients), negatively affected the respondents' evaluations of touch in therapy. Two factors, however, bear on the interpretation of this: (1) The sample in this study was composed almost exclusively of those with positive experiences of touch in their current therapy; and (2) the study did not adequately explore sexual attraction and seductiveness in the therapy dyad. This study did not ask whether a patient was sexually attracted to a therapist—a factor that might make touch "dangerous" or uncomfortable, even if a therapist has excellent boundaries.

CONCLUSION

Despite the overwhelmingly positive testament to the helpfulness of touch given by patients in their narrative answers, therapists need to proceed with caution when incorporating touch into their repertoires. Geib's (1982) parameters for using touch in psychotherapy, though strongly supported by the present research, are far from simple guidelines. They require astute clinical judgment, vigilant monitoring, and above all, sincerity and openness between therapist and patient. It is obvious that the patient's reaction to touch cannot be understood outside of its context, which in this case is the therapy relationship. Positive responses to Geib's factors and to the WAI both bespeak a high level of constructive involvement, cooperation, and communication in the therapy relationship.

As therapists we must also take into account our own histories and innate temperaments. A therapist who is not comfortable using touch should make it clear to a patient that this is a personal preference and/or a theoretical stance, so that the patient is not shamed by his or her need for physical reassurance or comforting. Both the therapist's and the patient's personal style, preferences, and expectations of therapy must ultimately be negotiated.

Obviously, the more cognizant we are of our own and our patients' needs and preferences regarding physical contact, the less likely it is that therapy will be aborted or stalled by misalignment in this sensitive area. Rigid rules prohibiting physical contact (or the converse, ritualized hugging) interfere with the rich opportunity to explore the varied feelings, self-perceptions, and interpersonal issues that are evoked by touch, touch hunger, or touch avoidance.

As Frank (1957) points out, language never completely supersedes the more primitive form of communication, physical contact. Touch can negate, reinforce, or otherwise alter verbal messages. Although it is impossible to separate the contribution of touch from the contributions of other aspects of the therapy relationship, many patients indicated that touch reinforced their sense of their therapists' caring and involvement, and that this allowed them to open up and take more risks in therapy. The results of this study thus support the judicious use of touch with patients who manifest a need to be touched, or who ask for comforting or supportive contact. They also confirm Ferenczi's (1953) position that, contrary to orthodox opinion, "gratifying" a patient does not necessarily interfere with the patient's motivation to work in therapy; indeed, it may alleviate shame and help the patient tolerate the pain enough to face and work through issues more quickly, or on a deeper level.

ACKNOWLEDGMENT

This chapter is based on my doctoral dissertation submitted in partial fulfillment of the requirements for the PhD degree at Georgia State University, 1994. The results of this study were previously published in Horton, Clance, Sterk-Elifson, and Emshoff (1995). Copyright 1995 by the American Psychological Association. Adapted by permission.

REFERENCES

Abbey, A., & Melby, C. (1986). The effects of nonverbal cues on gender differences in perceptions of sexual intent. *Sex Roles, 15*(5–6), 283–298.

Alexander, L. B., & Luborsky, L. (1986). The Penn Helping Alliance Scales. In L. S. Greenberg & W. M. Pinsof (Eds.), *The psychotherapeutic process: A research handbook* (pp. 325–366). New York: Guilford Press.

Bachelor, A. (1991). Comparison and relationship to outcome of diverse dimensions of the helping alliance as seen by client and therapist. *Psychotherapy, 28*(4), 534–549.

Bordin, E. (1976). The generalizability of the psychoanalytic concept of the working alliance. *Psychotherapy: Theory, Research and Practice, 16*, 252–260.

Ferenczi, S. (1953). *The theory and technique of psychoanalysis.* New York: Basic Books.

Frank, L. (1957). Tactile communication, *Genetic Psychology Monographs, 56,* 209–255.

Geib, P. (1982). The experience of nonerotic contact in traditional psychotherapy: A critical investigation of the taboo against touch. *Dissertation Abstracts International, 43,* 113A.

Gurman, A. (1977). The patient's perception of the therapeutic relationship. In A. Gurman & A. Razin (Eds.), *Effective psychotherapy: A handbook of research* (pp. 503–543). Elmsford, NY: Pergamon Press.

Hartley, D., & Strupp, H. (1983). The therapeutic alliance: Its relationship to outcome in brief psychotherapy. In J. Masling (Ed.), *Empirical studies of psychoanalytic theories* (Vol. 1, pp. 1–37). Hillsdale, NJ: Erlbaum.

Heslin, R., & Alper, T. (1983). Touch: A bonding gesture. In J. M. Wiemann & R. Harrison (Eds.), *Nonverbal interaction* (pp. 47–75). Beverly Hills, CA: Sage.

Hollender, M. (1970). The wish to be held. *Archives of General Psychiatry, 22,* 445–453.

Hollender, M., & Mercer, A. (1976). Wish to be held and wish to hold in men and women. *Archives of General Psychiatry, 33,* 49–51.

Holroyd, J., & Brodsky, A. (1977). Psychological attitudes and practices regarding erotic and non-erotic contact with patients. *American Psychologist, 32,* 843–849.

Horton, J. A., Clance, P. R., Sterk-Elifson, C., & Emshoff, J. (1995). Touch in psychotherapy: A survey of patients' experiences. *Psychotherapy, 32,* 443–457.

Horvath, A. O., & Greenberg, L. (1986). The development of the Working Alliance Inventory. In L. S. Greenberg & W. M. Pinsof (Eds.), *The psychotherapeutic process: A research handbook* (pp. 529–556). New York: Guilford Press.

Horvath, A., & Greenberg, L. (1989). Development and validation of the Working Alliance Inventory. *Journal of Counseling Psychology, 2,* 223–233.

Hubble, M., Noble, F., & Robinson, S. (1981). The effects of counselor touch in an initial counseling session. *Journal of Counseling Psychology, 28*(6), 533–535.

Lowen, A. (1967). *The betrayal of the body.* New York: Macmillan.

Luborsky, L., Crits-Christoph, P., Alexander, L., Margolis, M., & Cohen, M. (1983). Two helping alliance methods for predicting outcomes in psychotherapy: A counting signs versus a global ratings method. *Journal of Nervous and Mental Disease, 171,* 480–491.

Marmor, C. R., Horowitz, M. J., Weiss, D. S., & Marziali, E. (1986). The development of the Therapeutic Alliance Rating System. In L. S. Greenberg & W. M. Pinsof (Eds.), *The psychotherapeutic process: A research handbook* (pp. 367–390). New York: Guilford Press.

Marziali, E. (1984). Three viewpoints on the therapeutic alliance: Similarities, difference, and associations with psychotherapy outcome. *Journal of Nervous and Mental Disease, 172,* 417–423.

Mintz, E. (1969). On the rationale of touch in psychotherapy. *Psychotherapy: Theory, Research, and Practice, 6*(4), 232–235.

Nguyen, J., Heslin, R., & Nguyen, M. (1975). The meaning of touch: Sex differences. *Journal of Communication, 25,* 92–103.

Pattison, J. (1973). Effects of touch on self-exploration and the therapeutic relationship. *Journal of Consulting and Clinical Psychology, 40*(2), 170–175.

Robertiello, R. (1974a). Addendum to object-relations technique. *Psychotherapy: Theory, Research, and Practice, 11*(4), 306–307.

Robertiello, R. (1974b). Physical techniques with schizoid patients. *Journal of the American Academy of Psychoanalysis, 2,* 361–367.

Salvio, M., Beutler, L., Wood, J., & Engle, D. (1992). The strength of the therapeutic alliance in three treatments for depression. *Psychotherapy Research, 2*(1), 31–36.

Shepherd, I. (1979). Intimacy in psychotherapy. *Voices, 15*(1), 9–15.

Stein, N., & Sanfilippo, M. (1985). Depression and the wish to be held. *Journal of Clinical Psychology, 41*(1), 3–9.

Stockwell, S., & Dye, A. (1980). Effects of counselor touch on counseling outcome. *Journal of Counseling Psychology, 27*(5), 443–446.

Tyson, C. (1978). *Physical contact in psychotherapy.* Unpublished doctoral dissertation, University of North Dakota.

Wilson, J. (1982). The value of touch in psychotherapy. *American Journal of Orthopsychiatry, 52*(10), 65–72.

INSIGHTS FROM PRACTICE

10

THOUGHTS ON USING TOUCH IN PSYCHOTHERAPY

Joen Fagan

Her reason for wanting to see me for therapy wasn't flattering: She lived a few blocks away from my office, so she wouldn't have to cross any county or city boundary lines to get to me. I quickly found that agoraphobia was only one of her fears. She arrived late and out of breath to her first appointment, because she couldn't take the elevator and had to walk up the 11 flights of steps to my high-rise office.

She hadn't always been like this, she assured me. She had been a crackerjack legal secretary. Assigned to one of the rising stars of the law firm, she had begun an affair with him, which led to marriage and her resigning to become a housewife and hostess. This ideal relationship was inexplicably being ruined by her increasing withdrawal and growing number of fears. Her husband, she was pleased to report, was supportive but understandably exasperated. She had tried one therapist who had invited her husband in for a session. Wasting no time in demonstrating the therapist's incompetence and deriding him for his "touchy-feely" approach, the husband had declared he would never again go to a therapist with his wife, but certainly wanted her to do whatever was necessary to overcome her increasingly evident character flaws.

Reading between the lines left me grateful not to be on the witness stand with this attacking courtroom attorney trying to discredit me as an expert. It was clear that the intelligence and support my patient had provided him at the office did not transfer to home, where her limited middle-class background had not given her the skills to be the sophisticated hostess and glamorous escort that her husband desired. So in the first year of their marriage, his accurate, critical statements had shredded her self-respect until her world felt entirely too much for her to handle. No growth, ambition, expansion, or anger was possible.

I saw my tasks as demystifying her experience and offering her support for tentative ventures back into the world. Slowly, she was able to leave the house and spend time with friends. A year into therapy, she was faced with her husband's announcement of a new affair and a wish for a divorce. The financial settlement was adequate but not generous, and we were able to keep her grief and self-recrimination brief. At the 18-month mark, she started talking about going back to work. However, her self-doubts created big hurdles. She was sitting a few feet away, her hands flopping limply as she described being blocked by her expectations of failure. I leaned forward, tapped the back of one hand a few times with my index finger, and said, "These aren't helpless hands." She shrugged and switched to another topic for the remaining few minutes of the session.

During the next few weeks, almost every session was marked by reports of forward movement. She was thinking about going to law school; she had written for information; she had gone down to the school to get information; she was applying; a former college professor had encouraged her and written a strong letter of recommendation. I was delighted with this steady evidence of goal-directed growth, and was not surprised when she came in to say she thought she could leave therapy. I agreed that we had done well.

Several years later, I saw her by chance at a meeting. We found a private spot where we could talk, and she told me of having completed law school and of having found a job that she liked very much. She was living with a man, but was not yet certain if she wanted to marry him. She then said, "I've thought a number of times of calling you and letting you know what really happened that led to my stopping therapy. After you touched my hand, I was *furious*—'How dare you touch me!' I was so angry at you that I decided, 'I'll show you! You can't treat me like that!' So that started me on the road to law school. I'm sure now that it was a good thing, but I couldn't tell you at the time that that was that. I wasn't going to let you have the chance to treat me like that again. So I left—and did well." She smiled and extended her hand to me, said "Thank you," and left.

I went home and reflected on this surprising information. I had no idea what my simple gesture had tapped. In that moment of physical contact, had I become the mother who had slapped her hands in punishment, a bully on her playground who had poked and prodded her into misery, or her husband using his index finger to emphasize one of his devastating points? Whoever I was, the anger that had never been appropriately directed at the critical husband (or anyone else) used this ostensibly benign and supportive gesture by me to burst forth as a self-affirming and motivating force. It was just as well that she had not voiced her feelings at the time. An apology from me might have reduced her intensity; insight about the original source of the anger might have deflected the energy needed to propel her on her upward path. So, unaware, we had colluded on an elegant provision of the impetus to move her back into living.

This example serves as a reminder of the powerful and often unexpected effect of touch in therapy. Touch, like fire, can be a provider of light, warmth, nurturing, and movement, or of damaging and destructive consequences. After millennia of experience, we have largely tamed fire by providing many safety rules and devices, with fire departments as backup. Can we do the same with touch and make good use of its values while keeping its difficulties under control?

By the same token, a fire that does not catch and light offers its own problems. While I was a young, scared, self-doubting psychologist, I knew I needed therapy. I chose a man I had overheard at a professional meeting responding warmly to another person. However, after I had started as a patient, I felt a sense of needing more encouragement, support, and emotional reaching out than he was providing; still, he was the sophisticated therapist and I the naive patient who could only believe that he was doing it right. One day I went in to therapy crushed. Whatever had happened had left me in deep mourning. He said I looked like I was sitting *shiva*. That felt right, so I sat on the floor by his chair. Badly needing contact, I reached for his hand, which was resting on the arm of his chair a few inches away. He neither moved away nor responded, and I was left holding a lifeless imitation of a human hand. My ability to go into the deep feeling and release that I so badly needed was aborted, and I knew at that moment that I would get little of what I needed from him.

In my own practice, in individual therapy, I have never touched about one-third of my patients. With another third, I use touch as an affirmation of the relationship (e.g., I may hug a patient) or as a therapeutic technique (e.g., I may put my hand on a patient's back to help with the expression of grief, provide physical limits to help with anger expression, touch a patient to help evoke old memories, etc.). I have held another third of my patients extensively, as I would an infant or young child, as part of reparenting. I cannot remember more than a handful of experiences with touch that turned out badly; most often these came either when I moved too quickly without enough information or relational base, or when the permission I had requested before touching had been given by the patient with underlying reservations. Although strong feelings at times were evoked by touch, as in the example with which I have begun the chapter, these could be made therapeutically useful.

In addition, my experience has included teaching, training, and supervising many hundreds of aspiring and practicing therapists over 35 years. I have also directed several doctoral dissertations on touch communication (see Chapter 5, this volume). So I have had to do considerable thinking about the use of touch in therapy, as well as the great number of related issues. In the rest of this chapter, I would like to outline my views on the general kinds of touch, as well as on both the prerequisites and the reasons for using touch in therapy. Then I would like to spend some time looking at the fears (both external and internal) that go with this way of making human connection.

KINDS OF TOUCH

Touch is necessary to assist us in becoming human beings. Touch is the first language we learn—the one that defines our relationship to our mothers, provides pleasure, helps calm the storms of infancy. From the ways we were touched, our body egos develop—that is, our feelings about and perceptions of our bodies, and our comfort with touching and being touched. Absent or angry touch during our first years has dire effects. (In Chapter 5, I suggest that emotional and relational deficits accompany a lack of understanding of the meaning of touch communications.)

Touch is a very powerful language, with many more personal and idiosyncratic meanings than verbal language. To touch someone involves coming closer than the standard foot or two of space that we generally leave around ourselves and respect around others; intruding into that space almost always has significance. There are several kinds of touches, ranging from the public and formalized to the intensely personal:

1. *Ritual.* Ritual as touch may consist of a handshake, a victory hug, a pat on the back, or a "high five." The purpose of this type of contact is to affirm relational connections and roles, and/or institutional values.

2. *Athletic.* Athletic touch is the type that occurs in the course of

a contact sport (wrestling, football, etc.). The purpose is to display one's skill and best the opponent.

3. *Punishing.* Punishing touch includes slapping, physical abuse, and restraint. Here, someone who is literally or authoritatively bigger intrudes on another's body space to "teach a lesson" and to provide a discharge of emotion—usually anger.

4. *Nurturing.* Nurturing touch includes all kinds of good child care. For adults, it involves a voluntary letting someone into body space for general care (e.g., massage, beauty parlor services) or for treatment of particular problems (e.g., medical exams and procedures). The assumption is made that the service giver is benign and skillful.

5. *Intimacy-evoking.* This type of touch includes holding hands, cuddling, and the like, both to reinforce or increase intimacy and to give pleasure.

6. *Sexual.* Good sexuality involves personal pleasure and also can affirm intimacy by providing caring attention to one's partner.

However, especially as we move to the middle and end of this list, we find that many meanings and needs can be hidden under the obvious ones. Sexuality in particular can contain many other purposes and messages. For some women, the real goal of sex may be getting some kind of nurturing or intimacy. For a few individuals, sex may be used to punish, dominate, or fulfill personal agendas far removed from simply meeting sexual needs, as in rape or abuse.

PREREQUISITES AND REASONS FOR USING TOUCH IN THERAPY

If touch for most people contains many problematic aspects, these can become magnified in therapy. Very few of our patients were lovingly and appropriately touched by parents and others of significance. In general, the role of the therapist is often ringed by fantasy for the patient, who gives him or her a much-larger-than-life significance (this being partially necessary in the service of healing) filled with unfinished business. So the combination of need, fantasy, problems, and ambiguity stirs up old wounds. In my earlier example, for instance, a simple touch evoked a very strong response that was neither predictable nor visible. Touch opens up old, tightly closed doors to very early experience—which is nonverbal, often filled with emotional needs and expressions, and frequently surprising, but also potentially healing. So, even with a good history that gives us some knowledge of possible trouble spots, and with clear current consent, we still often do not know *whom* we are touching.

The basic prerequisites for use of touch in therapy, then, are these: clear therapeutic need; an adequate base of relationship and prior trust; explicit and ongoing permission; and (as much as possible) the patient's knowing what needs to be accomplished. Good training and experience, with supervision available are other essentials. A further necessity is the therapist's own clarity about physical contact, in order to provide as clear a field as possible. Before a therapist touches a patient, the therapist needs to be comfortable with his or her own body; to understand the differences among the different kinds of touches; to have his or her own nurturing and sexual needs met outside of therapy; and to be absolutely certain that ritual or nurturing touch is not an entrée to sexual touch and that there will never be sexual contact with patients. Finally, the therapist needs to be very clear about limits in general and to have carefully examined possible countertransference. *Touch should meet the needs of the patient, not the therapist!*

Given the considerations above, a partial list of reasons for a therapist to use touch in psychotherapy includes the following:

1. To prevent injury to self or the patient, or to prevent destruction of property.
2. To solidify the therapeutic relationship.
3. To help overcome a patient's specific deficits in experiencing emotion or in communicating with touch.
4. To evoke or intensify emotional states, such as to facilitate grieving or anger.
5. To increase the patient's body awareness, such as awareness of tension.
6. To evoke past emotional states and/or trauma.
7. To facilitate reparenting.

FEAR, AVOIDANCE, AND CONFUSION CONCERNING TOUCH

In spite of the many values of touch, insurance companies, licensing boards, training institutions, and individual therapists are presently all displaying large amounts of fear, avoidance, and confusion in regard to touch. A recent article by Gottlieb, Hampton, and Sell (1995) illustrates the confusion. The authors conducted a survey of practicing psychologists about how severely state licensing boards should treat offenders. They presented nine vignettes to be rated for severity, two of which involved simply "embracing" a patient after a treatment session to be supportive, or an "affectionate embrace" given in greeting a year after the patient's termination. Yet these were described as "cases of *sexual misconduct*" (my emphasis).

The parameters of touching which should be part of every therapist's training, are seldom included in such training. Therapists who are still willing to use touch are aware of being caught between a perception of the needs of patients and the potential large cost of any misjudgment. It is probable that national organizations such as the American Psychological Association, or training institutes that use touch as part of their work, could put forth training suggestions and protocols for touch. For example, in such guidelines, there would be a descriptions of appropriate uses of touch, problems that a therapist who touches patients might expect, ways to avoid these, and demonstrations of ethical decision-making processes about touching.

Finally, therapists' own anxieties may make touching patients problematic. Therapists have just as difficult a history with touch as anyone else. If their own therapy and training experiences have not addressed this, they have had only the standard corrective human experiences to give them help. So touch can bring up a variety of ill-defined or misunderstood old issues for therapists, including internal prohibitions, feelings of awkwardness, and even envy that they can give patients the loving touch that they themselves need. Some of the issues can be seen in the massive professional fear of "dependency," which is regarded as one of the worst things a therapist can evoke. What does this really mean? That the therapist doesn't know how to handle a needy patient, may not set appropriate general limits, or may be overwhelmed? It is true that in North American culture, one of our predominant values is that of "independence." Boys should be tough; young adults should leave home promptly; job promotions involving frequent moves are good even when families and friends are left behind; and sex is often portrayed in books and movies as solely in the service of physical needs, rather than involving relational needs. I suspect it is because of such cultural values and confusions that clear discussion, training, and guidelines about either dependency or touch are not available. Since this territory is not known or adequately explored, it is presumed to be dangerous beyond exploration—even as unknown territory was on medieval maps, which labeled it "Here there be Tiggers."

It is interesting and problematic that some of the last human frontiers are those closest to home. Therapists—both because of their own fears and their involvement with the fears of everyone else—are the ones who must struggle with issues of touch and dependency at the same time that they are punished for doing so in this increasingly adversarial legal and cultural environment. Because of that, their patients and society in general are deprived of the potential healing that a more open and permission-giving climate would facilitate.

REFERENCE

Gottlieb, M. C., Hampton, B. R., & Sell, J. M. (1995). Discipline of psychologists held in violation for sexual misconduct. *Psychotherapy, 32,* 559–567.

AN INDIVIDUALIZED AND INTERACTIVE OBJECT RELATIONS PERSPECTIVE ON THE USE OF TOUCH IN PSYCHOTHERAPY

Cheryl Glickauf-Hughes
Susan Chance

Almost 20 years ago, a psychology intern told her supervisor that her client had asked for a hug in their last session. She didn't know what the appropriate response was, and she asked the supervisor for advice. The supervisor told her that she had two good options: She could hug the client and process it, or not hug him and process it (M. Wells, personal communication, 1980). Implicit in the supervisors's response is the assumption that hugging a client is not an unethical act. The difference between touch with clients and touch with friends is that in therapy, we are committed to understanding the meaning of it for our clients.

Since then, psychotherapy has become increasingly dominated by fear of lawsuits (particularly lawsuits against therapists for sexual misconduct) and concern about managed care. Decisions regarding touch in psychotherapy are made far less casually than in the example given above. In some lawsuits or complaints to the licensing boards involving allegations of sexual misconduct by therapists, clients' boundaries have clearly been violated. In others, however, we believe that ethical therapists who use nonsexual touch as a common aspect of treatment may have done so with clients in whom such behavior has inspired feelings of longing and rage—and, as a consequence, fear and perhaps poor clinical judgment in the therapists.

For example, one therapist who often used body therapy as a component of treatment used these techniques with a sadomasochistic borderline client, who initially presented as much higher-functioning than she actually was. The client told her therapist that he was causing her to have erotic feelings, and she started to call him at his home. The therapist became uncomfortable, as this client had litigious proclivities; he abruptly stopped using touch in treatment. The client, feeling abandoned, terrified, and enraged, begin to call the therapist as much as 20 times a night. The therapist was unable to manage the primitive acting out of this client. Afraid that the client would sue him for sexual misconduct (she did not), he abruptly terminated his treatment of the client.

We believe that such a case exemplifies the use of touch with the wrong client, rather than a demonstration that touch is either unethical or uniformly "bad" for clients. The problems associated with using touch with this client were exacerbated by the therapist's rejecting behavior and his fear of being sued for sexual misconduct. In this chapter, we would like to suggest potential guidelines for touch in therapy, based upon the characterological styles of clients. These are intended to help therapists make thoughtful decisions about whether to use touch as a component of treatment with a given client.

HISTORICAL PERSPECTIVES AND CURRENT TRENDS

The majority of psychoanalytically oriented clinicians oppose the use of touch in psychotherapy (Freud, 1936; Strachey, 1934). According to these writers, clients transfer the feelings and yearnings they held toward significant individuals in their past, particularly parents, onto the therapist. This transference phenomena allows the client's previously unconscious or hidden feelings to become immediate and conscious and, therefore, available for exploration and understanding (Greenson, 1967). Psychoanalysts contend that the resolution of transference through insight and working through is the curative factor in psychotherapy (Freud, 1912/1958). They consequently believe that the needs and longings that are stirred in psychotherapy and become evident in the transference motivate the client to do the work of therapy. Thus, gratifying a client's wishes removes the tension necessary for the development of the transference and decreases the clients motivation to understand his or her experience.

Psychoanalytic theory is based on the assumption that childhood disappointments cannot be remedied by symbolic parenting later in life but must be accepted and grieved. Psychoanalysts such as Ferenczi (1919) who deviated from classical psychoanalytic techniques such as abstinence and believed that the use of touch in psychotherapy could be reparative were considered "wild psychoanalysts."

With the advent of humanistic and experiential forms of psychotherapy in the 1960s, therapists deemphasized the role of transference in treatment (Corlis & Rabe, 1969) and began to utilize more active approaches during psychotherapy. In the service of eroding formidable defenses and increasing the client's awareness, the careful and conscious use of touch was considered an acceptable psychotherapeutic intervention (Corlis & Rabe, 1969; Forer, 1969). Like Ferenczi, Mintz (1969) thought that a strict avoidance of physical contact could potentially repeat a physical rejection from the client's parents.

Recently, Norcross (1987a, 1987b, 1993) and others (Proschaska & DiClemente, 1982, 1984; Wachtel, 1994) have discussed the value of an integrationist approach to psychotherapy that allows clinicians increased flexibility in selecting theories that best fit his or her personality style as well as the client's (Norcross, 1993). In addition, there is a growing interest in the notion of tailoring the interpersonal stance of the therapist to best fit the needs of a given client (Beutler & Consoli, 1993; Dolan, Arnkoff, & Glass, 1993; Glickauf-Hughes & Wells, 1995, 1997; Lazarus, 1993; Mahrer, 1993; Norcross, 1993). This is in line with empirical data which suggests that the therapeutic relationship is the most important predictor of therapy outcome (Norcross, 1993). We believe that object relations theory provides a useful bridge between traditional psychoanalytic approaches and humanistic theories as it emphasizes the importance of understanding the etiology of the client's character as well as the importance of the here-and-now relationship between the therapist and client. In the remainder of the chapter, we will discuss an individualized and interactive object relations approach to the use of touch in psychotherapy.

OBJECT RELATIONS THERAPY

Until recently, the emphasis in object relations theory has been on theories of personality, development, and psychopathology. Although changes in treatment approaches have been suggested, only lately have theories of psychotherapy based upon object relations principles been explicitly described by such theorists as Cashdan (1988), Glickauf-Hughes and Wells (1995), Kohut (1971, 1977), Horner (1991), and Scharff and Scharff (1994).

Glickauf-Hughes and Wells (1995), in particular, believe that insight into unconscious conflict is necessary but not sufficient for change. They maintain that in addition to cognitive and even emotional understanding, clients require a corrective interpersonal experience—an actual demonstration that the world is different from what they have come to believe.Glickauf-Hughes and Wells thus emphasize several treatment goals, including (1) mastering unresolved developmental issues, (2) developing a more flexible and adaptive interpersonal style, and (3) developing more mature psychic structures. We discuss each of these in turn.

The first of these treatment goals is the mastery of unresolved developmental issues. Each client is viewed as having more or less successfully mastered the various phases of development that all people experience including basic trust, autonomy, separation/individuation, and initiative. To the extent that this process is incomplete—in other words, significant others didn't help a particular client resolve a developmental stage—psychotherapy potentially provides that client with a developmental second chance to do so.

The second goal of object relations therapy, as Glickauf-Hughes and Wells see it, is to help clients to develop a flexible and adaptive interpersonal style. Leary (1959) conceptualized individuals' behavior as potentially falling into one of four interpersonal quadrants (i.e., friendly–dominant, friendly–submissive, hostile–dominant, and hostile–submissive). To the extent that an individual's behavior falls exclusively within one of these four quadrants, and he or she is unable to switch to a different mode of relating when necessary (e.g., masochistic patients, who primarily behave in a friendly–dominant way, have great difficulty being friendly–submissive or hostile–dominant when it is appropriate), the individual's behavior becomes nonadaptive. Therapy thus becomes a place to learn new ways of relating to others that are less predetermined and more situation-specific.

Finally, in object relations therapy, a third goal of treatment is the solidification of a client's psychic structures. This includes helping the client develop the following: a cohesive sense of self that is differentiated from objects; an integrated sense of the various and sometimes incongruent aspects of the self; a strong ego that is capable of self-observation and good reality testing; and a sense of object constancy (i.e., a predominant positive internal object that the client can rely upon for a sense of security and self-esteem).

Thus, from an object relations perspective, the answer to the question "To touch or not to touch?" depends upon the therapist's assessment of the characterological issues of the individual client, including the client's attachment style, developmental impasses, and level of ego development and object relations. This assessment of the client's functioning and underlying dynamics influences what the therapist determines would be a corrective experience for that client, including whether or not touch would be a useful component of that experience.

CLIENTS FOR WHOM TOUCH IN PSYCHOTHERAPY CAN BE USEFUL

Unbonded Clients: Use of Touch to Develop an Attachment

Attachment or bonding occurs between parent and child before a child has the use of language, including receptive language. Thus, children learn to bond or attach to people through nonverbal communication— through eye contact, through attunement to the children's needs, through mutual nonverbal cuing, through smiling, and through touch. Harlow (1961) found in his experiments with infant monkeys that contact comfort led to attachment behaviors, whereas feeding did not.

Thus, when parents responsibly tend to an infant or child's physical needs but do so in a mechanical fashion, failing to provide the child with warmth and affection, the child often becomes detached, withdrawn, and emotionally unrelated to others. Without intervening corrective experiences from significant others in the child's life, the child usually develops into an adult who may function competently in many areas of his or her life but has chronic difficulties making meaningful attachments to other people. Individuals whose character is based upon this developmental failure are commonly referred to as "schizoid." Schizoid individuals often have the following characteristics. Generally, they are introverted and have a rich fantasy life that substitutes for actual relationships with other people (Guntrip, 1969). They thus have few if any relationships, and tend to feel detached in those that they have.

Guntrip (1969) believed that as people were not originally a source of nurturance for the schizoid individual, he or she learned to withdraw from others. Fairbairn (1952) described schizoid individuals as people whom love has made hungry; because they fear devouring the object with their hunger, they consequently shut their hunger off. Johnson (1985) observed that in addition to being detached from people and their own emotions, schizoid individuals often show little interest in eating and other life processes. It is thus common to find that schizoid individuals have overcathected intellects. Such people live in their heads rather than in their bodies. They tend to contact the world through their ideas, and pursue mental processes as a safe haven from relationships with people (Guntrip, 1969).

At times, however, diagnosing and treating schizoid clients can be confusing as such a client may have developed a seemingly socially adept false self that "acts" involved in the world. An important diagnostic cue for the therapist that there may be an underlying disorder of attachment is the therapist's frequent experience of feeling disengaged from the client himself or herself. We have found that for individuals who might be described as having schizoid proclivities, nonverbal relating that includes touch can be a useful and even a necessary component of treatment.

For example, one schizoid client, though superficially socially adept, was interpersonally remote and disengaged from her emotions to the point of inducing sleepiness in the therapist (who was otherwise somewhat of an insomniac). The client noticed the therapist's sleepiness; and the therapist initially explained it as a result of her own busy schedule, but processed the impact upon the client. After this pattern continued for months, the therapist noted that she did not become sleepy with any other client. The therapist thus began to process her own feeling of disengagement from the client, who talked about how disengaged she felt herself. The client also noted that she frequently had memories from her childhood of her mother sleeping on the couch and of feeling utterly unable to get the mother's attention. As this client's appointment was late in the evening, the therapist suggested that perhaps they should switch to an early morning appointment when the therapist was most alert and the client would have the highest probability of getting good attention.

The switch in appointment times made a dramatic difference in the client's level of engagement. Furthermore, the therapist began a ritual of bringing coffee into the session (prepared the way that the client liked it). The therapist noted that this also improved their alliance. She further noted that perhaps the most important component of the coffee ritual was the warmth of the coffee, which the client frequently commented upon. The therapist asked the client whether in general she experienced a lack of warmth in her life. The client talked about the lack of affection between her and her husband whom she experienced as even more remote than she was. The therapist asked whether this was similar or different from the state of affairs in her family of origin, and the client said that it was very similar—that neither parent was physically demonstrative.

The therapist began to observe that when this client experienced and talked about difficulties, she became increasingly intellectual, withdrawn, and inconsolable. After about 6 months of treatment, the therapist asked the client during a similar process whether she would like to try an experiment. She suggested to the client that she continue to talk to the therapist about the problems that she had been experiencing, but that she do so with her head on the therapist's lap. When the client did so, she began to express her problems with more emotions, began to cry, and said that she felt much better at the end of the session. Before she left, the client asked the therapist for a hug. Asking for a hug at the end of sessions became a fairly frequent occurrence, particularly during those sessions when the client felt particularly connected with the therapist.

In general, the therapist observed that the change in appointment time, the introduction of coffee, and the use of touch greatly increased the client's attachment to the therapist, and subsequently the client's attachment to other people in her life. In therapy (unlike the friendships), however, the meaning of these changes was always processed and understood. Furthermore, touch was not introduced into treatment until the therapist had a sufficiently good diagnostic understanding of this client's level of ego development and object relations functioning to be reasonably certain that an intervention such as inviting the client to put her head on the therapist's lap would not promote what Balint (1968) called a "malignant regression." Such a regression may occur in a tenuous therapeutic relationship, during which the client loses his or her capacity for self-observation; the regression is aimed at gratification by an external object, and the demands placed upon the therapist are intense, needy, and unrealistic. Such a regression did not occur in this case. Touch for this patient helped her to bond with or become genuinely engaged with the therapist, who was perhaps the first person with whom she felt this. It did not inspire an unhealthy dependence, symbiotic longings, or self-destructive acting out.

Neurotic/Overly Cognitive Clients: Use of Touch to Increase Spontaneity and Ability to Live in the Present

According to Glickauf-Hughes and Wells (1995, 1997), Kernberg (1975) and Wells and Glickauf-Hughes (1993), clients who have a neurotic level of ego organization and object relations development have the following characteristics. First, they have a clear sense of self and identity, and are able to differentiate themselves from other people. As such, close relationships with others do not cause them to feel engulfed and make them fear the loss of their sense of self-cohesion. Second, such clients have a sense of object constancy; that is they have an internal, primarily positive object upon which they can rely for feelings of comfort and security when other people are not present. Although they may feel lonely when they are by themselves or sad when they lose relationships with significant others, they do not experience decompensation, extreme separation anxiety, terror, and emptiness.

One type of neurotic character, the obsessive–compulsive personality, has been described as having a sense of rigidity, a lack of spontaneity, difficulty being playful, problems living in the present, an overcathected intellect, and a corresponding disconnection from emotions and sense of formality in relationships with other people. In general, obsessives prefer being right or in control to having good relationships with people.

Although touch is not as important in overcoming significant developmental problems with obsessive clients as it is with schizoid clients, we have found that the judicious use of touch—particularly in the middle phase of treatment and in groups—can at times be extremely effective in the psychotherapy of these clients without causing damage to them, as it might with clients who have a borderline level of ego organization and object relations development.

For example, one group client tended to obsess and to remain intellectual when speaking in group about his troubles, making it difficult for people to be helpful to him. Sometimes he asked the group for advice—which he of course rejected. The therapist helped him become aware of his propensity to avoid feelings and his difficulty getting help from other people for fear of giving up control. However, insight didn't seem to have an impact upon this process. After this client had been in group therapy for approximately 7 months, the therapist asked him during one session (when he was ruminating in the group and losing the attention of the group members) whether he knew what he needed from the group. Whereas previously he would have said "advice," he was aware at this stage that advice wouldn't really be helpful to him. He thought about the therapist's question and said that he didn't really know what he needed. The therapist then asked him whether he would be willing to try an experiment. He said that it depended upon what it was. The therapist suggested that while he continued to talk about his problem with his boss, perhaps someone in the group would volunteer to massage his shoulders. He said that he felt a little bit awkward, but that he would try it. As the other group member began to touch him, he began to relax and stopped talking.

He laughed and said that maybe talking wasn't what he needed. He continued to have his shoulders massaged while the next client worked. After the next client finished, the therapist returned to the first client and asked him how he felt, and he said that he felt much better. Through this process the client became more aware of what he needed from other people, learned the limits of getting his needs met through talking, and eventually learned to use talking in a way that was more helpful to him (i.e., he became less cognitive, more direct, more emotionally expressive, and more able to be vulnerable).

A second important use of touch with obsessive clients is to increase playfulness. Obsessive clients tend to approach life in a deadly serious manner. Although their defenses are not primitive, they generally have a lot of them, and these tend to be quite rigid. We have found that the use of touch in a playful way helps bypass defenses and increases obsessive clients' sense of spontaneity. Furthermore, it tends to evoke less shame than does the use of humor. Thus, such gestures have been used with clients who were stuck in a struggle with their therapists, themselves, or other people. On one occasion, a therapist lightly threw a pillow at a client. On another, she gave him a playful, light punch on the shoulders (in the manner in which men often demonstrate affection to one another). On a third occasion, she gave a client a bear hug. Each instance was followed by laughter and a temporary dissipation of defensiveness or of a struggle for control.

Counterdependent Clients: Use of Touch to Make Dependence Needs Ego-Syntonic

For a number of character types, primarily oral and masochistic/self-defeating characters, normal dependence needs have become ego-dystonic or shameful (Glickauf-Hughes & Wells, 1995). Such individuals' parents were responsive enough to them as infants, enabling them to make an attachment to others. However, the parents were generally rather immature and undependable; they also commonly manifested significant problems, such as alcoholism, bipolar disorder, and borderline or narcissistic personality disorder. As such, in these parent–child dyads the parents' needs took prominence over the children's needs. Such children were often shamed for their needs and told that they were in some way "too much" for the parents. In contrast, they were tremendously reinforced for taking care of their parents' needs, through which they got their own needs met vicariously. This pattern of parentification and overdetermined caretaking of others is often a socially reinforced one, especially for women. As such, it frequently continues through the individual's adult life.

Although such individuals are usually quite aware of the needs of others, they are often unaware of their own needs. For example, one client worked at two jobs, ate her lunch in the car, came home and made dinner for her husband, and then spent several hours on the telephone solving the problems of her friends. She noticed that she was overeating and gaining weight, and that she felt depressed but she didn't understand why.

When such individuals are aware of feeling needful, it is perceived as a global state, and they experience a great amount of shame about feeling it. For example, one group client asked for time, said that she felt "bad," talked more than usual, and felt ashamed afterward. In fact, such clients believe that just having needs will make people reject them and thus make them less likely to get their needs met. This client consequently avoided eye contact with other group members while she was talking.

Thus, such clients develop a number of defense mechanisms for dealing with the awareness of normal needs. The first is denial. For example, one client stayed so busy that she had no awareness of her needs, even her hunger.

The second defense is projection. Thus, when one client was feeling unloved, she would go out and purchase special presents for her husband and friends. Such clients often project their needs onto others and then try to meet the others' needs. Sometimes they guess correctly. For example, the client who was unaware of her needs but spent many hours on the phone with her friends understood that what her friends needed was attention, concern, and being understood. Sometimes, however, they do not guess correctly. Thus, for example, during one couple therapy session, a husband who was very doting with his wife and rarely asked her for anything touched her throughout the session "because she was having a hard day." In actuality, she found his touching her to be intrusive. When she had a hard day, what she desired was time by herself to unwind. The therapist processed this dynamic and asked him whether he perhaps needed affection from her at that moment.

Unfortunately, none of these defense mechanisms solves the problem of getting normal needs gratified and accepting an important aspect of oneself. In fact, the chronic caretaking of others generally leaves one more needful. However, such individuals do not tend to be structured at the borderline state of object relations and ego development. Therefore, techniques such as the use of touch, which enable them to bypass defenses and become more aware of needs and feelings, are generally not detrimental to them.

One of the ways touch can be important to such a client is that it simultaneously enables the client to become aware of a need and to have the need gratified. The impact is often radical. In addition, the use of touch can help underline the client's resistance to feeling needs and feeling dependent upon another person. For example, one group member with these dynamics asked one of the other group members to massage her shoulders. While this was occurring, she begin to speak in an intellectual, fast, overly contained manner. The therapist asked her how it felt to have the other group member massage her shoulders. She said that she was aware that she wasn't feeling anything. When the therapist explored this with her, she said that she felt afraid to relax and trust someone to soothe her, as she believed that good experiences always turned into bad ones. The therapist asked her whether she had any associations to this, and she remembered a time when her piano teacher had affectionately stroked her hair when she had played especially well—and then suddenly "whacked me on the back of the head with no explanation." She then began to talk about the level of violence in her home, particularly in regard to her father's behavior toward her mother. She became aware that she associated nurturing touch with abuse.

Finally, masochistic clients are generally structured at the preneurotic level of ego and object relations development. Clients at this level have a cohesive sense of self and have differentiated self and other, so there is no danger that touch will induce a loss of self-cohesion. However, such clients have incomplete object constancy, as they have failed to internalize the soothing and empathic functions of caretakers; indeed, their caretakers were often abusive. Because of their difficulty in self-soothing, it is important not to rely too heavily on touch as a means of soothing these clients, as touch is more difficult to internalize than, for example, empathy and the provision of auxiliary ego functions. Consequently, overrelying on touch for soothing, rather than using it at moments to break down a barrier and provide the clients with the visceral experience of being comforted, can be infantilizing to these clients: It can lead them to believe that they require the actual presence of the therapist in order to feel good. Such a belief can lead to an unhealthy regression.

Thus, there are a number of clients for whom touch can be a powerful tool for increasing awareness; overcoming resistance and rigid defenses; and mastering the developmental phases of attachment, dependence, and trust. In all cases, however, ego development is presumed to be sufficient, so that touch induces what Balint (1968) called a "benign regression." Such a regression is characterized by (1) a mutually trusting relationship; (2) maintenance of observing ego functions; (3) the recognition and working through of internal problems; and (4) minimal demands upon the therapist. Clients in whom touch induces a malignant or untherapeutic regression are discussed next.

CLIENTS FOR WHOM TOUCH IN PSYCHOTHERAPY IS ADVISED AGAINST

Clients Who Use the Therapist as a Permanent Solution Rather than as a Bridge to Mature Relationships

Not all clients come to therapy for treatment (Glickauf-Hughes & Wells, 1997). Rather, they may unconsciously come to repeat a trauma, to prove that the world is not trustworthy, or to experience the happy childhood they feel entitled to but never had. When therapists become aware that they are treating clients in this category, particularly clients with a borderline level of ego organization and sadomasochistic tendencies, they are advised not to use touch as a part of treatment. This is often difficult, as such clients frequently request physical gestures such as holding from their therapists, and continue to request it as a means of testing limits when the therapists say no.

For example, early in her career, one of the us was treating a high-functioning borderline patient (i.e., one with a stable work history, only one brief prior hospitalization, and only moderately self-destructive acts—she binged on ice cream, but spit it out rather than ingesting and vomiting it). After about 4 months of treatment, the patient asked the therapist for a hug at the end of a particularly meaningful session, and the therapist granted her request. The next day, the client called the therapist with an emergency four times. The therapist scheduled an appointment with her the following day.

When the client's affective state was processed, it appeared as though a number of issues were evoked for her by the use of touch. The first was a sense of longing and wish for symbiotic merger with the therapist. The other was a fear of merging with the therapist and losing her sense of self. After noting and processing the impact upon the client of touching the therapist, the therapist made the assessment that touch in therapy was not in this client's best interest, and explained to her why she believed that. The client initially accepted, this but frequently solicited physical affection from the therapist and felt wounded when the therapist processed rather than gratified her wish. The client also initiated inappropriate touch with the therapist (e.g., running her fingers through the therapist's hair as she was leaving the office). This extended to other activities that pushed boundaries, such as refusal to leave the therapist's office after sessions, leaving notes on the therapist's car, and following the therapist around the grocery store.

For clients such as this one, we believe that the use of touch makes the boundaries between therapist and client unclear. It also inspires unrealistic longings (such as the wish for symbiotic merger) that get acted out through extreme testing of limits and suicidal gestures. Thus, for most borderline clients, we have found that touch generally inspires a malignant regression, including the feeling of entitlement to have a good childhood and relentless attempts to use the therapist for this purpose. We have found that therapy generally proceeds better with such clients when touch is not used in the first place. Such limits actually serve to contain the clients' longings and fears.

Clients with Engulfment Issues

As discussed earlier, there are individuals whose parents, because of their own impairment, were not able to facilitate the children's developing a secure attachment in which other people could be reasonably depended upon to meet their needs. In contrast, other clients' parents enabled their children to learn to bond adequately, but were threatened by the separation/individuation process (Johnson, 1987). For example, clients with narcissistic parents, who tend to develop narcissistic issues themselves, were not allowed to individuate (i.e., to develop and mature in ways that reflected their true natures). Rather, the parents required the children in some ways to be what the parents wanted.

In some cases, a child was expected to be an ideal parent to the parent (i.e., one who was empathic, soothing, and admiring). For example, one client was regarded by her mother as her best friend. When the mother experienced problems with her alcoholic husband, she frequently used her child as a confidant. The client remembered often holding her mother when she was crying, and also recalled her mother's holding her to soothe her when the mother was feeling needy.

In other cases, a parent needed a child to be the parent's ideal self. Thus, one obese mother who wished to be beautiful controlled her daughter's appearance, including putting her on diets and having her lift weights from an early age. She had her daughter modeling and performing in plays, and devoted one whole wall of the house to pictures of her performances. When this client looked through family albums, she could find no pictures of herself "playing like a regular kid." Another thing that struck this client when viewing family albums was that although she remembered (and still experienced) her mother as cold and unaffectionate, in family pictures her mother frequently put her arm around her or had her pose by giving her mother a kiss. Affection was thus experienced as something that was used to create a public impression.

In either case, a child was never accurately seen. Such a parent tended to touch the child when the parent, rather than the child, felt needy; to ignore the child when the parent was not in the mood but the child was needy; or even to wake a sleeping child to show him or her off to friends. Such individuals thus become hypervigilant as adults about being used by others. Because their needs (including needs for touch) were never attended to by parents, they are often quite unaware of these needs themselves. Affectionate gestures, including ones by the therapist, are consequently interpreted as efforts to "use" such a client in some way and are often experienced as impingements. For example, the wife in the couple therapy session discussed earlier (see "Counter-dependence Clients," above) disliked her husband's affectionate gestures, as she sensed that they were really a way of getting his own needs met under the guise of meeting her needs. This experience was a recapitulation of the infantilizing and smothering affection that she received from her mother.

It is thus advised that for a client with clear narcissistic issues, fears about being used, or fears of having boundaries impinged upon, the therapist should be very circumspect and cautious about the use of touch—particularly in the earlier phases of treatment, when transference of the impinging parent is still very salient. Sometimes at later stages of treatment with such a client when the true self with its awareness of needs and feelings is better developed, the use of touch can be slowly introduced. Even then, however, it is best done in response to the client's initiative.

Clients with a History of Poor Family Boundaries (i.e., Sexual Abuse Survivors)

Sexual abuse survivors are not a homogeneous group (Wells, Glickauf-Hughes, & Beaudoin, 1995). They vary greatly in both character style and level of ego development. As such, Wells and colleagues believe that treatment for these clients is variable and contingent upon a number of factors (e.g., development of object constancy, level of ego strength). Nonetheless, when it comes to making treatment decisions regarding the use of touch with these clients, several principles are frequently applicable. These include the following:

1. If the therapist has any reservations at all, it is best to forgo the use of touch.
2. Touch is almost always not appropriate in the beginning of treatment.
3. Initiation of touch should usually come from the client.
4. When touch is initiated by a sexual abuse survivor with a borderline level of ego organization, and the therapist notes a strong countertransference response, it is very important for limits to be set and for the therapist's response to be processed.

Thus, for such a client, the therapeutic alliance needs to be clearly established and the transferential fear of being used and abused needs to be worked through before touch can be beneficial. The cue for touch must always come from the client, and touch optimally begins within a context that makes sense and seems appropriate (e.g., the client's asking the therapist for a hug at the end of a particularly meaningful session, after trust has been built between therapist and client).

However, it is important to note that when touch is initiated by the client in a manner that disrespects the therapist's boundaries and makes him or her feel uncomfortable, this usually indicates that some sort of projective identification is occurring. For example, the border-line client discussed earlier who ran her fingers through the therapist's hair and refused to leave the office had been sexually abused as a child. The therapist shared with the client that the client's behavior made her feel uncomfortable and invaded. She then asked the client whether that was how she had felt as a child, and the client begin to discuss her feelings about being sexually abused as a child.

SUMMARY

The answer to the question "To touch or not to touch?" is not simple. Therapists who endure rigid theoretical assumptions and consistently use forms of treatment that never or always include touch save themselves the considerable struggle of making individual decisions with each client.

We believe, however, that touch in psychotherapy is useful to some clients and not to others. In this chapter, we have tried to outline some guidelines that we have found helpful in making treatment decisions in this area. These include (1) not using touch with clients who have a more primitive level of ego organization and object relations development, as in such cases it frequently promotes a malignant or unconstructive regression; (2) using touch cautiously and in response to the clients' request with individuals who have been used (particularly in a sexual manner) by parents; and (3) using touch more frequently with higher-functioning clients whose core issues are inability to bond, shame about needs, and lack of awareness about feelings and needs.

Finally, this list is not intended to be conclusive. Rather, it is meant to be a starting point for therapists to conceptualize their own guidelines for the appropriate use of touch in psychotherapy.

REFERENCES

Balint, M. (1968). *The basic fault: Therapeutic aspects of regression.*. London: Tavistock.

Beutler, L., & Consoli, A. J. (1993). Matching the therapist's interpersonal stance to client's characteristics: Contributions from systemic eclectic psychotherapy. *Psychotherapy, 30,* 417–422.

Cashdan, S. (1988). *Object relations therapy.* New York: W. W. Norton.

Corlis, R. B., & Rabe, P. (1969). *Psychotherapy from the center: A humanistic view of change and growth.* Scranton, PA: International Textbooks.

Dolan, R. T., Arnkoff, D. B., & Glass, C. R. (1993). Client attachment style and the psychotherapist's interpersonal stance. *Psychotherapy, 30,* 409–412.

Fairbairn, W. R. (1952). *An object relations theory of the personality.* New York: Basic Books.

Ferenczi, S. (1919). Introjection and transference. In S. Ferenczi, *Sex in psychoanalysis* (pp. 35–57). New York: Basic Books.

Freud, A. (1936). Transference. In A. Freud, *The ego and mechanisms of defense* (pp. 18–25). New York: International Universities Press.

Freud, S. (1958). The dynamics of transference. In J. Strachey (Ed. and Trans.), *Standard edition of the complete psychological works of Sigmund Freud* (Vol. 12, pp. 97–108). London: Hogarth Press. (Original work published 1912)

Forer, B. R. (1969). The taboo against touching in psychotherapy. *Psychotherapy: Theory, Research and Practice, 6,* 229–331.

Glickauf-Hughes, C., & Wells, M. (1995). *Treatment of the masochistic personality: An interactional–object relations approach to treatment.* Northvale, NJ: Jason Aronson.

Glickauf-Hughes, C., & Wells, M. (1997). *Object relations therapy: An interactional approach to psychoanalytic treatment.* Northvale, NJ: Jason Aronson.

Greenson, R. (1967). *The technique and practice of psychoanalytic treatment* (Vol. 1). New York: International Universities Press.

Guntrip, H. (1969). *Schizoid phenomena, object relations and the self*. New York: International Universities Press.

Harlow, H. F. (1961). The development of affectional patterns in infant monkeys. In B. M. Foss (Ed.), *Determinants of infant behavior* (Vol. 1). New York: Wiley.

Horner, A. (1991). *Psychoanalytic object relations therapy*. Northvale, NJ: Jason Aronson.

Johnson, S. (1985). *Characterological transformation*. New York: Norton.

Johnson, S. (1987). *Humanizing the narcissistic style*. New York: Norton.

Kernberg, O. (1975). *Borderline conditions and pathological narcissism*. New York: Jason Aronson.

Kohut, H. (1971). *The analysis of the self*. New York: International Universities Press.

Kohut, H. (1977). *The restoration of the self*. New York: International Universities Press.

Lazarus, A. (1993). Tailoring the therapeutic relationship, or being an authentic chameleon. *Psychotherapy, 30*, 404–407.

Leary, T. (1959). *Interpersonal diagnosis in psychiatry*. New York: Ronald Press.

Mahrer, A. (1993). The experiential relationship: Is it all purpose or is it tailored to the individual client? *Psychotherapy, 30*, 413–416.

Mintz, E. (1969). On the rationale of touch in psychotherapy. *Psychotherapy, 6*, 232–234.

Norcross, J. (1987a). Commentary: Eclecticism misrepresented and integration misunderstood. *Psychotherapy*.

Norcross, J. (1987b). Introduction: Eclecticism, casebooks and cases. In J. Norcross (Ed.), *Casebook of eclectic psychotherapy*. New York: Brunner/Mazel.

Norcross, J. (1993). Tailoring relationship stances to client needs: An introduction. *Psychotherapy, 30*, 402–403.

Proschaska, J., & DiClemente, C. (1982). Transtheoretical therapy: Toward a more integrative model of change. *Psychotherapy, 19*, 276–288.

Scharff, J., & Scharff, D. (1994). *The primer of object relations therapy*. Northvale, NJ: Jason Aronson.

Strachey, J. (1934). The nature of the therapeutic action of psycho-analysis. *International Journal of Psycho-Analysis, 15*, 126–159.

Wachtel, P. (1994). Theory, practice and the nature of integration. In H. Arkowitz & S. Messer (Eds.), *Psychoanalysis and behavior therapy: Is integration possible?* New York: Plenum.

Wells, M., & Glickauf-Hughes, C. (1993). A psychodynamic–object relations model for differential diagnosis. *Psychotherapy Bulletin, 28*(3), 41–48.

Wells, M., Glickauf-Hughes, C., & Beaudoin, P. (1995). An ego/object relations approach to treating childhood sexual abuse survivors. *Psychotherapy, 32*(3), 416–429.

12

LONG-TERM CLIENTS' EXPERIENCE OF TOUCH IN GESTALT THERAPY

Suzanne Imes

The climate of our times is a litigious one, in which blaming others for one's losses, mishaps, or tragedies is commonplace. In this climate, there is an emphasis on power over others, rather than on personal power and responsibility. In response, many psychotherapists avoid touching clients for fear clients will sue them for sexual misconduct because they are angry about something else. On applications for liability insurance, some companies have begun asking therapists for justification if they touch clients.

I believe that touch should be available and allowable in therapy. However, I don't think it is necessary for all clients. I have personally been a client of one therapist who uses touch liberally in her work, and of another one who rarely touches physically. The former has helped heal the touch-deprived child in me. The second therapist has touched my body with her mind—with wise insights that find matching templates deep within me and seem to restructure my cells into their original essence.

I have some clients whom I rarely if ever touch, either because they have been too wounded to tolerate or trust touch, or because they were *not* extremely wounded or neglected. In contrast, I have worked with clients for whom touch was a pivotal aspect of treatment. I believe that clients themselves are the best resources for discovering if, when, and how touch is beneficial to the therapeutic process. They are the ones who can give us "justification" for using touch in psychotherapy.

Thus, although we therapists can theorize about what is important to clients, my goal for this chapter was to learn directly from clients about their experience of touch. In particular, I wanted to learn whether themes might emerge that might instruct me and other therapists in the use of touch in psychotherapy.

THE USE OF TOUCH IN GESTALT THERAPY

Gestalt therapy was the predominant therapeutic approach used with clients discussed in this chapter. The forms and use of touch in Gestalt therapy have been described extensively by Edward W. L. Smith (1985) and James I. Kepner (1987), so I will not attempt to explain these in detail here. In brief, within the framework of the Gestalt contact–withdrawal model, I use both "soft" and "hard" techniques. The contact–withdrawal model is based on the assumption that satisfaction in living involves cycles of making contact with people and things in one's environment, and then withdrawing from that contact. The model includes the two major aspects of awareness and expression. Awareness begins with a want, which leads to arousal, which leads to emotion. If none of these is stifled or inhibited, expression can take the form of action and interaction, and can end in satisfaction (Smith, 1985, pp. 35–37).

Smith (1985) defines psychopathology as *"any pattern of habitual self-interruptions in the contact/withdrawal cycles"* (p. 34, emphasis in original). Self-interruption can take place anywhere along the contact–withdrawal continuum through blocking arousal, clouding awareness, preventing action, and preventing appropriate interaction.

In deciding whether touch might be useful to a client, I watch and listen for where a client self-interrupts. The four tasks of the body-oriented therapist, according to Smith (1985), are to "facilitate aware-ness, facilitate breathing, melt body armor, i.e., stop retroflected action, and stop retroflected interaction" (p. 119). "Retroflection," in Gestalt terminology, is either turning back on the self what a person would like to do to someone else, or doing to oneself what one would like someone else to do. Thus, if clients are not aware of what they want or feel, I will look for an interruption in breathing that can inhibit arousal and energy to act. If the breathing is shallow or limited to the chest or to the diaphragm, I may ask permission to put my hand gently on the restricted area of breathing. This is an example of "soft" touch, which can help a client enhance awareness and access to the energy needed for the expression of a feeling or desire.

I used such a "soft" technique with a client[1] who habitually defended against feelings by staying in her head. I noticed that her legs and knees were clamped together like an oyster protecting its insides. I touched one knee lightly to bring attention to her retroflected energy and asked, "What would happen if you let your knees fall apart?" She did this and immediately began crying. Afterward she was aware of how she "held tears in her legs" and was able to express her sadness when she felt safe enough.

A client whose feelings are less accessible may benefit from the use of a "hard" technique, which may involve deep pressure at an area of the body where there is extreme spasticity, or "body armoring." Melinda was such a client, who complained often of tightness in her lower back. She asked me to press hard into that area. As I pressed, she began moaning and had images of her father molesting her as a child. Although she had already worked through many of her incest-related symptoms, Melinda reported that after working in this manner several times, she began for the first time to gain an interest in having sex with her husband.

John told me that he was angry at his boss but felt powerless to do anything about it. Neither his voice tone nor his facial expression gave any indication of the degree of the anger his words described mechanically. He had been beaten as a child, and had learned to inhibit his own anger for fear of being hurt even more if he expressed it. I could see tightness in the muscles of his jaw, in his shoulders, and in his legs—the body armoring he had used to inhibit his anger all his life. In the context of group therapy, where there were enough people to contain his anger without anyone's getting hurt, I suggested a "limits structure"—another "hard" technique, in which the person is held tightly and allowed to move and emote within the safe limits of others' providing a container for the long-held feelings. After John strained against the group members' pressure and yelled out his angry feelings toward his boss, the faces of his abusive parents replaced that of his boss, and he was able to express and release the anger he had felt toward them so long. With that backlog of anger released from his body, he could then decide on an appropriate course of action with his boss that was more congruent with the current situation.

In Gestalt therapy, we often suggest "experiments" to clients to enable them to complete either "unfinished business" from the distant or recent past, or unfinished situations from dream material. The experiment brings the situation into the present, where the client can use fantasy, words, and/or actions to complete the traumatic or unfinished event with a more satisfying or empowered outcome. Since people remember unfinished situations more readily and keep them more in the foreground than they do finished ones, the symbolic completion of a traumatic event allows it to recede into the background of a person's emotional landscape. Thus, with a sexual abuse survivor, I may hold up a pillow to represent the abuser and suggest that the client push the pillow and yell "Go away!" or "Stop!" or "Get out of here!" until she has the physical or emotional feeling of getting rid of or stopping the abuser who overpowered her in the past.

As the years have passed and I have gained ongoing training and experience with touch in therapy, the more likely I am to err on the side of caution and of interrupting the client's process with discussion about touching. For example, even in the midst of deep and/or regressed work, I might say, "Would it feel right for me to touch your jaw?" or "Let me know if my touching you in any way would help," or "Remember, if I touch you in some way that doesn't feel right, even by accident, say 'Stop, I mean it' and I will stop immediately." Such instructions, within the context of the Gestalt experiment, provide the client with a feeling of safety and of being in charge of any touch that might be included.

A SURVEY OF CLIENTS ABOUT TOUCH IN GESTALT THERAPY

To honor a client-centered approach to touch in therapy from the beginning, a group of clients was invited to participate in a focus group on touch in therapy. The clients were asked to think about what had been important to them about touch in therapy, and to generate questions most likely to tap into the relevant aspects of being touched by one's therapist. From that group discussion, a questionnaire was developed (see Table 12.1).

The questionnaire was given to trainees at the Gestalt Institute of Georgia,[2] to clients in group therapy, and to selected clients in individual therapy who I thought might help clarify the relevant issues in this area. I attempted to get information from clients who had been touched extensively, moderately, and rarely—in order to explore similarities and differences in their responses, as well as to discover what themes about touch might emerge.

Some of the following questions arose in my mind: What kinds of clients desire touch and respond very favorably to it? Which clients benefit from touch but don't feel a need for it? Which clients are resistant to touch or afraid of it? Who benefits from touch and who doesn't? What kinds of touch are beneficial for what kinds of clients?

TABLE 12.1. Touch in Psychotherapy Questionnaire

<u>Consent Form</u>

Edward Smith, Pauline Rose Clance, and Suzanne Imes are editing a book about the use of touch in psychotherapy. Suzanne is writing a chapter on long-term clients' experience with touch in therapy. Will you please help us gather the information we need by completing the enclosed questionnaire and returning it to your therapist as soon as possible?

If we include parts or all of your writings in the book, we will attempt to disguise particulars so that you cannot be identified, unless you let us know you don't mind being recognized. So please give us the demographic information below and sign your name to the agreement that suits you.

Name _____

Address _____

Day phone _____ Night phone _____

Sex _____ Age _____ Race _____

Length of time in therapy with the therapist you write about _____

Therapist's name _____

You have my permission to use the information in my questionnaire as I have written it, as long as you do not use my name or other obviously identifying data.

Your signature _____

You have my permission to use the information in my questionnaire, if you will change details in such a way that my identity is not likely to be recognized. I understand that you will get my approval before publishing any summary or direct quote of my account.

Your signature _____

You do not have permission to use any of my material except as a part of group data. No direct quotes.

Your signature _____

Thank you for your help.

Suzanne Imes, PhD
Licensed Clinical Psychologist

(*continued*)

TABLE 12.1. (*continued*)

Questionnaire

1. What is your history of touch in your family or origin? (Who touched whom, and how did that feel to you? How were you touched as an infant, toddler, grade-school child?)

2. Does your therapist use touch in your present psychotherapy?
   Never _____ Sometimes _____ Frequently _____

3. A. Was touch relevant in your choice of a therapist?
      No _____ Yes _____ Somewhat _____
   B. What has been your experience of touch in your present psychotherapy? (Please explain when and how your therapist touches you. In other words, what are the circumstances, conditions, or parameters of touch in your psychotherapy? Be specific.)
   C. Describe as fully as you can your personal experience of being touched in therapy.

4. What do you want your therapist to know about you and touch in psychotherapy?

5. What cues and/or information do you give about touch to your therapist? In other words, how do you let your therapist know how and whether you want to be touched?

6. A. Does your therapist convey to you that s/he will hold the boundary of not being sexual with you when s/he is using touch in psychotherapy?
      Yes _____ No _____
   B. How or how not?

7. A. Do you think touch is important in psychotherapy?
      Yes _____ No _____
   B. Why or why not?

8. A. What is helpful (or good) touch in psychotherapy?
   B. What is not helpful (or bad) touch in psychotherapy?
   C. How do you discriminate between bad and good touch in psychotherapy?

9. How has touch facilitated your process in psychotherapy?

10. How has touch interfered with your process in psychotherapy?

11. Do you think that touch or lack of touch in psychotherapy substantially contributes to the outcome of psychotherapy? Please explain.

12. How do you think your therapy would be different if you had not been touched?

13. What would you like to tell us about touch or lack of touch that has not been covered by these questions?

In organizing an approach to the rich and complex experiences that were reported, I noted that there seemed to be a relationship between clients' desire for and responsiveness to touch in therapy and their experiences as children. People could be roughly categorized into the following groups in terms of the extent that touch was used in working with them in therapy:

Extensive use of touch

1. Extreme sexual, physical, and/or emotional abuse during childhood
2. Touch deprivation during childhood

Moderate use of touch

1. Moderate physical and/or emotional abuse during childhood
2. Physical invasion during childhood
3. Adequate childhood touching and no abuse

Minimal to no use of touch

1. Extreme sexual, physical, and/or emotional abuse and/or neglect during childhood
2. Unmet dependency needs during childhood with little current environmental support

Overall Differences in the Use of Touch

Several overall differences were apparent in the clients with whom touch was used extensively, moderately, and minimally/not at all. The most obvious differences were in the degree to which the clients themselves wanted to be touched, and the extent to which they believed touch facilitated or did not facilitate their therapeutic process. Those differences corresponded roughly to the developmental stage in which the clients were traumatized and to the extent of their trauma. Those who experienced extensive abuse, neglect, or terror at an early age were the clients for whom touch was the most *or* the least beneficial. Clients in the moderately touched group experienced more trauma in the prepubescent or adolescent years; although people in this group often spoke glowingly of the benefits of touch, it did not have the life-saving quality for them that it often had for clients in the extensively touched group.

Touch involving holding or other "reparenting" approaches were used extensively with clients in the first group, as were "hard" touch techniques, which are useful in helping clients in accessing and releasing deep emotions held tightly in body armoring. The clients in this group often mentioned the nurturant, connecting, and humanizing value of touch. By contrast, touch was most often used in the context of Gestalt experiments with clients in the moderately touched group. These clients frequently stressed the value of touch in facilitating awareness and promoting expression of feelings.

Although some clients in the first group did not want to be touched in the beginning of therapy, they eventually sought out and valued many varieties of touch and experienced these as providing a safe container for them to do their work. The clients in the second group tended to remain more cautious about touch throughout therapy, stressing the need to "be in charge" of the touch, the importance of ongoing dialogue about touch with the therapist, and the importance of touch's not being used for the therapist's benefit or in any way that would interfere with the expression of the clients' feelings.

Clients' Views of "Good" and "Bad" Touch in Psychotherapy

The two clients who received minimal or no touch in therapy both stated simply that "good" touch is touch that is wanted and "bad" touch is touch that is not wanted. All the other clients agreed with this assessment in one way or another.

In both the extensively and moderately touched groups, there was general agreement that good touch is respectful of the client's wishes, is done for the benefit of the client and not the therapist, facilitates the therapeutic process, and is amenable to honest discussion. Bad touch is the opposite of these. All clients who had been sexually abused at any age added that bad touch is touch that feels sexual, or touch on any sexual area of the body; several clients who had not been sexually abused also included sexual touch in their definitions of bad touch.

Clients in the moderately touched group also stressed the importance of noninvasive touch and the importance of being "in charge" of whether or not the therapist touches them. Clients in the extensively touched group were more likely to emphasize the importance of being able to get the therapist to stop any touch that does not feel right to them.

CLIENT ILLUSTRATIONS

I have chosen a few clients who I think are representative of several of the categories listed above. For all but one of these clients, I have been the primary therapist; I therefore discuss my own experiences and thoughts about the process of touch, in addition to reporting from the clients' perspective. In all cases, touch was only one modality used within the overall context of ongoing, long-term therapy.

Extensive Use of Touch in Therapy

The two childhood experiences associated with extensive therapeutic use of touch were suffering extreme abuse or being touch-deprived. I discuss the former first.

Extreme Sexual Abuse during Childhood

Research on touch in psychotherapy is showing that people who were abused as children—especially those who were sexually abused—generally evaluate touch in therapy positively and believe that touch is beneficial in the process of working through the resultant legacy of shame, fear, self-loathing, and mistrust. In Chapter 9 of this book, Horton reports that 71% of her abused subjects (the majority of whom were either sexually abused or both sexually and physically abused) wrote that "touch repaired self-esteem, trust, and a sense of their own power or agency, especially in setting limits and asking for what they needed" (p. 132). Many learned that touch need not be sexual.

Since touch in therapy can be particularly beneficial to sexual abuse survivors, I have chosen to give in-depth accounts of the experience of touch in therapy of two of my long-term clients who were repeatedly and violently sexually abused by a parent from a young age. In reading their accounts, I myself have become more attuned to the extreme importance for the therapist of solid training in body-oriented therapies, acute sensitivity to verbal and nonverbal cues, and open and continuing dialogue with clients about their responses to touch.

Client 1: Ellen. When Ellen entered therapy with me 15 years ago, she had recently had one session with a therapist who had suddenly given her a "big bear hug" at the end of the session. About that event, she wrote:

> I was generally terrified and on the edge of psychosis. She could not have been reading my cues. I sat as far from her as possible, jumped with anxiety, and at other times sat rigidly and woodenly. Looking back, I can't imagine what possessed her to hug me. What it told me was that she would overwhelm me just like my mother, so I never went back.

I can imagine myself making the same mistake as that therapist did back then—a time when touch flowed freely in humanistic therapeutic settings, and when I myself had benefited profoundly from being touched as a client in therapy. Luckily, Ellen's negative experience with touch instructed us both. Touch is a form of intimacy, so touching too much too soon can feel inauthentic or intrusive.

I will never forget our first session. Not only was this affable, bright, articulate, and very frightened young woman able to tell me not to touch her, but she also proceeded to warn me about a host of other therapeutic approaches and techniques that would surely frighten her away from this venture. As I ran through her catalogue of prohibitions in my head, I realized that I would not be able to use much of what I had learned about being a psychotherapist. She could not tolerate anything in the therapist's repertoire—not reflective listening; not behavioral interventions; and, heaven forbid, anything as "techniquey" as empty-chair work. I smiled internally, with a deep respect for this person's integrity and resistance to anything that smacked of interpersonal inauthenticity. I must admit also to being worried about how in the world to be with her. However, my Gestalt training to be "in the now" and Ellen's ongoing honesty guided and stretched me, and taught me how to work with a severely sexually abused person.

Ellen had been violently sexually, physically, and emotionally abused from babyhood to adulthood by her apparently psychotic mother. Her experience was reminiscent of the abuse of Sybil, described in the book by the same name (Schreiber, 1973). Over time, numerous parts of herself emerged as she recalled incident after incident of her mother's treachery—from the tiny, terrorized, crying "Babies" to the 12-year-old "Bad Girl" to the teenaged "Cutter" and the adult "Shadow Man." Each part of herself had split off to cope with the various and unpredictable tortures of her mother.

Working with Ellen within the Gestalt therapy theory and perspective, I considered all of her "parts" valid and understandable introjects and adaptations to what was happening to her at the time of the abuse. At the same time, I tried to honor her skepticism about therapy. Ellen remembered the following about touch in her therapy:

> She did not attempt to touch me for several years. She then began offering end-of-session hugs, for a while used touch to help me differentiate between her and me, and later began using touch to facilitate feeling release (e.g., pressing my forehead), holding me when I cry, patting me to ground and/or calm me, etc. I think she also touched me to let me know that she was right there with me.

Regarding my use of touch to help Ellen differentiate between us, I had learned that her mother had so thoroughly taken possession of Ellen's body that she did not know where her mother stopped and she began. She transferred this lack of boundaries to me, often putting her mother's face on me, while at the same time developing a separate relationship with me as Suzanne. When I felt the bond of trust was quite strong, I began to talk with Ellen about what she fantasized it might be like for me to touch her arm lightly (a Gestalt experiment—using fantasy when the client cannot tolerate a hands-on experiment). After many discussions and much fantasizing, Ellen allowed me actually to touch her arm. At first she literally could not feel my touch, so thoroughly had she deadened herself to the dreaded touch of her mother. After many repetitions of this experiment, Ellen's skin cells began to "wake up" and warm up to a gentle, nonthreatening touch. She began to experience for the first time meeting another person at the contact boundary of her skin without fear.

In *Gestalt Therapy Integrated,* Miriam and Erving Polster (1974) explain the contact boundary as follows:

> What distinguishes contact from togetherness or joining is that contact occurs at a boundary where a sense of separateness is maintained so that union does not threaten to overwhelm the person. . . . The contact boundary is the point at which one experiences the "me" in relation to that which is not "me" and through this contact, both are more clearly experienced. (pp. 102–103)

Ellen's experience of touch as a child had left her confused about the difference between overwhelming fusion with another person and healthy contact. Through gradual, noninvasive touch in therapy, Ellen began to experience the rudiments of having a separate self. It was only much later that she could experience comfort and then pleasure in being touched.

Ellen recalled in her questionnaire that in the beginning of therapy she couldn't stand for *anyone* to touch her; she assumed that all touch was sexual. She went out of her way to avoid touch, but was able to warn close friends not to touch her. She wrote, "A big piece of the terror touch held for me was that I could not control or limit it—I had no power, was at the mercy of the other, and was absolutely alone and vulnerable." She noted that although she is still fairly reserved about touch until she knows someone well, and still cannot allow anyone to touch her sexually, she likes very much to be touched by people she knows well. She even feels touch-deprived from living alone, and she appreciates hugs.

To the question "What do you want your therapist to know about you and touch in psychotherapy?", Ellen responded:

> Safe, noninvasive touch is absolutely critical to my being able to do deep work. I am convinced I would not have been able to go to some of the inner places I've gone and faced the terror I've faced had she not been holding on to me, as this (1) let me know very concretely that I was not alone, (2) soothed me enough to go through it, and (3) grounded me enough in the present to keep a sliver of adult ego functioning so that, in the end, I always came back from the terror.

Ellen was the first client I worked with who had been sexually abused, and her therapy began before the proliferation of training workshops and literature on adult survivors of childhood sexual abuse. Thus, on the one hand, I was working in the dark with Ellen; on the other hand, my Gestalt perspective proved to be a good fit for relating to Ellen. I learned by listening and watching in the present as carefully as I could to her verbal and nonverbal cues, such as a subdued voice tone, darting eyes, or a very still body, all of which might indicate that she had begun having memories of a past trauma. I also worked extensively with the various disowned parts of herself in dialogue with each other and with people of her past, to complete unfinished business and to achieve integration.

I extensively used both regression and "presentification"[3] in my work with Ellen—going back into a past traumatic experience; reexperiencing the images, memories, and pain of a particular event; and calling on the part of herself that had dissociated at the time to construct a different outcome, such as screaming at her mother to go away, or imagining calling in people in her present life who could protect her from her mother. During such experiences, in addition to making sure she did not become retraumatized by remaining too long in her terror, I might touch her lightly just to let her know I was there, role-play her mother (with a pillow between us) so she could push her away, or hold the sobbing child who had never gotten comfort back then.

To the question about the importance of touch in therapy, Ellen responded:

> I could not have tolerated much of this process without touch. It has enabled me to get out of my head, go deeper, and heal a lot of touch-connected wounds, for example, seeing myself as untouchable and unlovable, equating any touch with sex, etc.

Because it had been Ellen's mother who abused her, I assumed that it would be especially important for me, as a woman, to make it quite explicit that I would never be sexual with her. I was later to learn that clients abused by men would also project their fear of abuse onto me; I needed to be just as forthright with them in vowing aloud never to be sexual with them, though I don't recall needing to reassure them quite as often or over such a long period of time. Ellen pointed out six ways she thought I conveyed that I would hold the boundary of not being sexual with her: (1) by telling her again and again, (2) by being clear about other boundaries, (3) by talking openly with her if she was worried something might be sexual, (4) by paying attention to body language and asking what was happening, (5) by always stopping any touching when she told me to, and (6) by being very respectful of her boundaries and only pushing gently.

In describing the difference between "good" and "bad" touch in therapy, Ellen emphasized the importance of (1) touch that avoids direct contact with sexual areas, (2) touch that she is in charge of (i.e., she can stop it when she wants), (3) touch that springs from her needs and not the therapist's, and (4) touch that facilitates the process she's in rather than stifling or impeding it.

Ellen reiterated in several ways in the questionnaire that "safe" touch in therapy helped her discriminate between sexual and nonsexual touch, and that it allowed her to heal touch-related wounds, such as seeing herself as untouchable and unlovable. She also emphasized that touch was critical in the overall healing process. She wrote:

> Touch communicates in a way that words do not and thus facilitates and speeds the process of healing. Touch says stronger than words that you are two real people involved in a real albeit professional relationship, and that makes it safer to explore deeply painful and even terrifying places within yourself. I think it would be difficult, if not impossible, to do deep feeling work without touch, and thus to make more than cognitive changes. [Without touch,] I'd still be dealing with (skirting) the same issues in the same old ways, rather than feeling pretty much healed on the cognitive, emotional, and even cellular levels. I am a completely different person than when I started therapy with this therapist. I think her judicious use of touch was absolutely essential in my healing. It provided a stimulus and a literal physical container for my feelings, and that helped me move through and out of them. I think that without touch, my wounds would have been bandaged but not healed.

Ellen's life is no longer dominated by what happened to her as a child; she no longer identifies herself primarily as a survivor of sexual abuse and she has terminated therapy. During the course of therapy, she earned a PhD and is now a well-respected professional in her field. All this was gained in the midst of doing extensive regressive work in individual therapy, group therapy, and numerous 2- to 5-day intensive workshops, where she bravely confronted and extirpated the demons of her past. As she reflected on the role of touch in therapy, she added the following thoughtful advice to therapists using touch:

> I think it's important that touch not be initiated by the therapist until (1) you really know the client and (2) have a solid relationship. In the beginning you should ask or offer touch before doing it, and make it clear that refusal is OK. Constantly processing the client's experience of touch (early on) short-circuits therapist pleasing as well as resistance. Regarding the criticism that touch fosters unhealthy regression and dependence: I think you can avoid/limit the "unhealthy" part by stressing the need for developing ways to get needs met outside of therapy and by focusing equally on the adult and child ego states. I think the danger lies in the therapist who is a little too gratified by the dependence, intensity, or whatever, and in the client who is not willing to take steps toward developing self-support, support outside the therapy, and responsibility for his/her life in the present regardless of what's happened in the past. You shouldn't use touch with that kind of client until that willingness is in place. Hence the need to know who you're dealing with before you initiate touch.

Client 2: Barbara. Barbara reminds me to be cautious about touching clients, especially clients who are doing a significant part of their therapy at a preverbal level. During the early years of her therapy, Barbara would often spend a portion of the therapy hour literally unable to talk. Because she was a successful attorney who was facile with words and who was able to interact quite "normally" with others in social situations, I initially sometimes mistook her silence for angry, passive resistance to therapy.

When I asked her to draw what she couldn't speak, it became apparent to both of us that being in the therapy setting allowed her to reenact the silent withdrawal into which she often escaped as a child, and which enabled her to confront images of abuse that she had previously avoided. Many of her drawings depicted a child and a penis. Finally she could tell me in a child's halting voice, "Daddy hurt."

I vividly recall Barbara's startle response whenever I made a gesture with my hand as I talked or reached up to scratch my nose. Her head jerked back reflexively, terror streaked across glazed eyes, and the rest of her body froze like a squirrel in the street facing an oncoming car. Efforts to reassure her that I would not hurt her were of no avail until I could match her stillness and quietly coax her into a more mature state of consciousness. At first, when I asked where she went when she was feeling scared, she could not remember and was not even aware that she had dissociated to numb her fright. Later she could explain that I looked just like her father, and she was scared that I would hit or molest her. Clearly, to touch Barbara at times like this would have terrified her further.

But it was not always so evident to me when touch would be useful and when it might create terror or rewounding. I was apparently responding to her own ambivalence. Barbara wrote about touch in her early years in therapy:

> I thirst for it, yearn for it, am terrified by it, judgmental of it, terrified that the therapist will hurt me, terrified that she will lose control of her boundaries, terrified that my boundaries would disappear, and I would become irretrievably psychotic.

Barbara never became psychotic. On the contrary, her courageous working through of her childhood terrors, including her fears about touch, has been transformational. "NOW I love touch," she wrote. "It tells me that I'm loved, it tells me that the relationship has intimacy, and it helps me do my work."

To the question "What do you want your therapist to know about you and touch in psychotherapy?", Barbara responded: "In early therapy, not to be fooled into thinking I am just yearning for it, but to also be aware of the fear." In person, I asked Barbara for examples of times I had not paid enough attention to her fear, in order to instruct myself and other therapists through my mistakes. She recalled a time about 9 years earlier when I moved toward her too aggressively in a role play simulating her father; she was terrified and frozen and couldn't tell me what she was feeling. On another occasion when she was in a regressed state, my thumb was too close to her mouth, and she was petrified, imagining my thumb to be her father's penis.

When therapists make inevitable mistakes with clients, it is important to acknowledge the mistakes and to initiate dialogue about the clients' responses to them. Barbara wrote that although sometimes touching made her feel terrified, or powerless, or out of control of the situation, "when this happened by mistake, having the opportunity to process this with my therapist was extremely important." This highlights the importance of asking clients frequently whether touch feels comfortable to them. If the client doesn't answer, I now ask for a nonverbal signal, such as raising a finger. If I still get no response, I believe it is important to stop touching until the client is able to talk.

In reply to the question "What cues and/or information do you give about touch to your therapist?", Barbara remembered that early in therapy she gave no direct cues,

> . . . because I had no idea or words about this, no observing ego to help me make any sense of my experience. I used to react very strongly to movements that were too fast or too strong, or if I didn't want her near me, I would make a palpable boundary of angry energy to protect me.

However, not all clients, especially those who have experienced life-threatening abuse, are able to produce the kind of "angry energy" that Barbara used to instruct me about the personal space that she needed to feel safe. As stated earlier, because of the compliance required of many abuse survivors as children, they may *appear* to be benefiting from or liking touch while they are inwardly cringing in terror.

Like Ellen, Barbara believed that "good" touch is "solely for the client's benefit" and is "done with the clear understanding that the client is ultimately in charge of the touch," with the therapist watching for verbal and nonverbal cues that indicate "no, stop, or enough from the client."

Although I have used Barbara's writings to caution readers about clear communication with clients in nonverbal states, I again do not want to instill inordinate fear about touching such clients. Despite her fear of touch, Barbara many times invited touch in the therapeutic work. She wrote:

> Body work, during feeling work and regressive work, acts as a bridge to my feelings. Holding has nurtured me. Hugs at the end of sessions communicated that I was OK, that my circumstances were not so abnormal that we couldn't partake in this simple human ritual. Touch has deepened my experience, thereby facilitating my movement in therapy.

She also stated that through touch her tactile yearning was fulfilled, and that touch was "nice help" when she couldn't talk much. In addition, she speculated that touch perhaps contributed to more direct, extensive healing, since she was damaged by touch.

Thus, the two survivors of sexual abuse I have described here felt that respectful, well-timed, noninvasive touch enhanced movement of the therapeutic process, made their feelings more accessible and expressible, communicated that they were valuable human beings, and provided a safe nurturing container in which they were able to work through terrifying memories. Not all sexually abused clients feel as positive about touch in therapy. This will be addressed later in this chapter.

Touch Deprivation during Childhood

When a baby is not held and cuddled, he or she is likely to grow up questioning his or her lovableness and right to exist. If that same child is later encouraged to perform and achieve, but receives little validation of his or her true feelings, the child is likely to grow up with an "as-if personality"—performing according to parental expectations on the outside, but feeling unworthy or empty on the inside (see Miller, 1981).

Client 3: June. June's is the story of a child who did not want to exist—the story of a girl who felt burdened from the outset of her life by a needy mother, an overworked, underpaid father, and a critical and dominating older brother. June was a child who longed for touch, but rebuffed her smothering mother, and had only minimal access to touch from her lovable but passive father. Nurturing, loving, and playful touch by her aunt and uncle when they visited are cherished memories. She was a beautiful, intelligent, sensitive, and talented child who used her gifts to develop the "as-if" personality that would gain her praise and approval for her "show," but little real sense of solidity or substance.

When June entered therapy at the age of 31, she presented her well-put-together self in designer business attire, makeup, and hairdo fit for the cover of *Working Woman* magazine. She spoke articulately about a recently ended relationship with a married man and about her lack of fulfillment in a challenging, lucrative, but unfulfilling career path.

One day, after a few months of dealing with these adult matters of relationship and career concerns, June impulsively crawled into my arms. She lay there like a baby bird fallen from its nest, outwardly still, but trembling on the inside. Her breathing was rapid and shallow, and her chest muscles and bone structure had the underdeveloped and fragile feel of a premature baby's. I often thought of her as a "preemie." For many months, the therapy consisted of talking to her a little at the beginning of the session, holding her for most of the rest of the session, and then helping her return to an adult state at the end. During these holding times, I found that my slow, steady breathing against her chest would deepen and slow June's breathing and calm the internal trembling. Not only was I modeling deep, slow breathing for her to follow, but I was also "lending" her the sound of my heartbeat, which she told me had a calming effect on her. For a long time, she could not find any words to connect with her experience or feelings while she was being held.

Although I wondered if such partial reparenting would be enough, I believed that June knew best what she needed. I predicted that it would pay off in the long run, for several reasons: (1) My own experience as a touch-deprived client with a therapist who was comfortable holding me had been quite healing; (2) June had a healthy support system outside of therapy; (3) she always "came back" to an adult state at the end of the therapy hour; and (4) along with calming touch and deeper breathing came less depression and more strength in June's outside functioning (i.e., touch was not creating an unhealthy regression). She was, for example, able to change to a more satisfying job and to end periodic dating relationships that didn't feel right to her.

June described her experience of touch in therapy as follows:

> My therapist began to touch me as a part of psychotherapy approximately 3 or 4 months after I started therapy. Primarily, for the first 2 years, she held me and focused my attention on my breathing while having contact with her body. Therapy equaled being held for quite some time. The circumstances and conditions for the particular type of body therapy I was receiving was that I would come in, we would talk for a short period of time, and then either she or I would initiate the physical contact.
>
> There was very little talking in the sessions during that time. The parameters included being held with the therapist's whole body. While being held, I was allowed to touch her face, hair, or skin on her arm. It was never spoken, but I understood the rules. After a period of time, body therapy took a variety of forms. It included the therapist using her body to create resistance for me to push against, placing her hand on my upper chest or back to release emotional pain locked in those areas of my body, cradling my neck in her hands, or touching painful areas on my body so I could make internal contact between my mind and body.

As she experienced more contact between her mind and body, June became more "real." She spoke and acted more out of her authentic feelings and needs, rather than out of her perception of other people's expectations. Much of her reluctance to express her true self arose from her deep-seated shame about her neediness for love, affection, and nurturance. As is often the case with people deprived of early nurturance, June experienced her neediness physiologically as a painful hole in her chest:

My experience of therapeutic touch was that it provided a medium for me to get in touch with very old pain and longings. When I started psychotherapy, I had pains around my heart area and an imagined space inside my chest that felt like a gaping hole. When I would experience the pain and hole inside my chest, I would become extremely depressed. As I held on to my therapist, I was unable to speak, and could only focus on the sensation in my chest. At the end of each session, once separated from her, I could physiologically feel the difference in my chest. It felt full and refreshing. However, it took a long time for that sensation to stay with me for more than a day. All the contact in therapy felt good, and the longer I worked at a physiological level, the better I felt. Outside of therapy, I enjoy touching. I have had mostly positive experiences being touched. I have never been invaded physically, so I don't have any fears about it. Since I have done the body work at such a deep level, I have found that I don't long for touch as much as I used to, and subsequently do not initiate it as much.

Although therapy can never totally erase the damage caused by early lack of nurturance, June's experience shows that touch in therapy can be significantly reparative. She was able to internalize the feeling of safety and security afforded by touch, gradually gaining more self-support and depending less on the external support of therapy:

Touching helped me feel connected to my own body and to my therapist. It has been a life saver for me and was the underlying catalyst that allowed me to do deeper work on my own. It provided a secure base I never experienced internally before. Because of the extensive work I have done, when I am hurting or scared, I can mentally transplant myself back in my therapist's arms and feel myself breathing. The internal contact and focus on my own body calms, nurtures, and puts me in a meditative state. It helps me to get through very hectic days just by stopping and breathing. I trusted, loved, and learned a great deal from my therapist and through touch in psychotherapy. It opened up new choices for me that did not previously exist.

Some of those new choices have included entering into a loving committed relationship, deciding on a new career path, and nearing the completion of a doctorate in her chosen field. June only comes to therapy now for periodic "check-ins," and it is a delight to see how a radical approach to touch in therapy has helped this "preemie" develop into a grown woman of substance—one who is more fully alive, is no longer depressed, and expresses a great enjoyment of love and work.

Moderate Use of Touch in Therapy

Either Moderate Abuse or Adequate Touching during Childhood

The responses I received from clients indicated that moderate use of touch, usually in the context of Gestalt experiments, had been positive particularly for clients whose childhood experience fit into one of two categories: either moderate physical and/or emotional abuse, or adequate childhood touching and no abuse. Their needs were much the same as those reported by others in terms of wanting touch to be respectful, noninvasive, and nonsexual. In general, touch was not as emotionally "charged" for them, either positively or negatively, as it was for people in the other groups. I have not included cases from these two groups.

Physical Invasion during Childhood

People who were physically invaded as children, however—that is, those who experienced physical intrusion from adults (e.g., poking, pushing, or other unwanted touch)—presented some special needs in regard to touch. These are illustrated below in the discussions of Laura and Joe.

Client 4: Laura. Frankly, I was surprised when I read Laura's account of her experience of touch in psychotherapy. During the course of her 10 years of individual therapy, 7 years of group therapy, and participation in several intensive workshops, I have heard more about how Laura doesn't like to be touched than about how she does. I have exercised great caution about touching her; even with such vigilance, I have assumed I must have made enough mistakes along the way to contribute to Laura's apparent view of touch as primarily negative. But to the question of her personal experience of touch in therapy, she replied:

> What comes to my mind immediately is warmth. The circumstances in which my therapist touches me are always to convey love and warmth. My personal experience with touch has been extremely important and helpful. Physical touch by my therapist has helped me get in direct contact with my emotional experience. Touch has added a dimension to my therapy that has deepened my therapy and awareness at a visceral level.

Laura described touch in her family of origin as "mostly intrusive," with her mother and father "poking me, hitting me in the face, pulling or pushing me." No one in this family of six hugged anyone else or touched with warmth or caring. Laura remembered all touch as being violent in nature, and said that "touch does not feel safe to me." Although her father was not directly sexually abusive, he sometimes asked Laura to touch him in ways that felt somewhat sexual to her, and she therefore did not trust his sexual boundaries. Thus, touch in therapy has not always felt safe because of her family history with touch. However, Laura has been able to speak clearly about her current feelings about touch, especially in the context of group therapy, where she has been able to compare her reactions to touch with those of others in the group.

Unfortunately, *I* have not always been as cognizant as I might have been about the connection between Laura's current fear of touch and her negative experience with touch as a child. I learned through the questionnaire that, in addition to helping her heal by "deepening feeling release and grief work," experiencing touch in therapy has also helped her be more assertive in saying what doesn't feel OK, and it has helped her learn that "no one knows what is best for me but me." Because Laura is a very psychologically sophisticated client, my lack of cognizance was not damaging; with a less insightful client, however, I might have missed an opportunity to help the client verbalize and anchor such learnings.

The themes of boundaries and choice are especially salient for Laura and appear several times in her questionnaire. In response to the question "What do you want your therapist to know about you and touch in psychotherapy?", she wrote: "With my history it is very important that I have a choice about touch. I was invaded a lot in my family, so for it to be OK not to be touched is important." She considers "helpful" touch to be touch that is "intended to heal," that is "respectful of the client's boundary," and is "wanted, not done to you." Unhelpful touch, according to Laura, is that which "is not associated with the client's needs/boundaries," and "touch that hasn't been invited or a therapist who doesn't ask to touch certain areas of the body."

Laura had experienced an unintended touch error with another therapist. It was important that she was able to express her grievances on this occasion, and that the therapist who erred was nondefensive. But there was also a positive side to the touch error for Laura. She had held the view that a therapist should always be able to meet a client's needs and should never make mistakes. Through the process of resolving this and other "betrayals," she learned a great deal about living through disappointment, not depending on others always to "get it right" for her, and forgiving herself and others in all their humanness.

Client 5: Joe. Although I have never been Joe's primary therapist, I have known him for a long time—many years ago as a client in group therapy, and more recently as a participant in Gestalt training. His questionnaire responses refer to his 13 years of individual therapy with a male therapist of the experiential school, and to group therapy with that same male therapist and a female Gestalt therapist.

Joe, like Laura, was physically invaded as a child; Joe was particularly invaded as a teenager by his mother, who would crawl into bed with him in the mornings to wake him up. He described his family as "huggy" and liked his father's "bear hugs," even though the father seemed a little "uncomfortable" with hugging. Although Joe's childhood experience with touch in the family got mixed reviews, in contrast to Laura's totally negative report, Joe was even more adamant than Laura in his emphasis on choice and boundaries. When he wrote about end-of-session hugs with his individual male therapist, he noted how important it had been to exercise the choice not to hug when he didn't feel like it, as well as to be able to talk with his therapist about not wanting to hurt his feelings if he said "no" to touch.

Both touch and the absence of touch have allowed Joe "to learn about personal boundaries . . . setting them for myself, that others can respect them, that relationships do not disappear when I set them." According to Joe,

> Good touch is supportive, is used with talk, is given when needed and requested, is used with permission. Bad touch is for the therapist's sake only. Bad touch would be sexual or invasive in other ways. And it is touch that is not given with permission, even if the intentions are good.

Also, Joe wrote of his strong belief that "there should always be discussion about the touch (not necessarily right away or during) so that the patient's 'adult' is engaged."

In group therapy, Joe has sometimes experienced touch by other group members "at a sensitive moment" as interfering with his process. This raises an interesting question for those of us who do group therapy: Should we interrupt if one member moves to touch another without clear permission? When I have had qualms about the timing or appropriateness of touching, I have at times, for instance, said to a toucher, "You might ask Suzy [Jim] if she [he] is OK with your touching her [him] right now," or, to a person being touched, "Pay attention to whether you're wanting to be touched right now, and let John [Jane] know." In such a way, we can possibly help clients become more aware of their own and other people's touch boundaries, and we can let them know that explicitly asking and telling are both important aspects of an interactive process.

Joe wrote that there were times when he allowed touch by one of his therapists when he didn't want to, in order to "please" the therapist. On these occasions, he walked away feeling that he had betrayed himself. Coming back and talking with the therapist about such incidents strengthened their relationship. "But I could imagine," Joe warned, "some people coming in and not being able to say no, so therapists must be very sensitive to this." This further supports the importance of therapists' periodically checking out their clients' experience of touch and making it easy for clients to discuss motivations such as "therapist pleasing."

Joe described his touch with his male therapist as an indicator of advances in therapy: "Getting gradually more at ease with each other has allowed touch to advance." With his female therapist (a Gestalt therapist who uses touch as part of her therapy), on the other hand, Joe noted that "touch has in fact been an important part of advancing the therapy." He described some touch experiences with her:

> Sometimes pressing on my shoulders has allowed me to access feelings more fully, such as anger or burdened. Or touching and pressing my chest over my heart has allowed me to feel more deeply and completely sadness and hurt, allowed feelings to move through me so I felt better, became less stuck. She even climbed on top of me during a "feeling release" session, mimicking my mother's invasiveness. This was a brave and delicate thing she did, but I remember it, and it paid off, because it increased my awareness and helped me feel better.

Joe ended his description with another cautionary note:

> Please remember, however, that I have also had many years with her, and so trust has built up to where I could let her do what she did and be OK with it. I would not have wanted to do this early in our relationship.

To the question "What cues and/or information do you give about touch to your therapist?", Joe replied that he is now usually able to tell his therapists if he wants touching. Sometimes he uses body language (e.g., folding his arms or sinking back in his chair if he doesn't want to be touched). Sometimes now he asks one of his therapists to sit next to him in group or just goes and sits by one of them. "It has come to be mostly a playful experience," he noted, "whereas earlier in therapy it may have felt more serious a decision." In the questionnaire, the theme of developing trust over a long period of time emerged often for this client who was repeatedly invaded physically as a child.

On the other hand, there were times when Joe wanted to be touched but didn't ask for fear of "being greedy or selfish to want so much." Although I have already said a great deal about using caution in touching, it is also important to be sufficiently attuned to clients that touch is occasionally provided when a client can't or doesn't ask for it. With clients whom I do not know well, or with whom touching parameters have not been clearly established, I may say something like this: "You look like you could use a hug. Is that right or not?" or "I wonder if it might help you access your grief if I put some pressure on your chest?" or "Would it help if you came over and sat by me or someone else in the group?" I hope that such questions invite rather than invade, and give the client a chance to say yes or no. If a client says an immediate yes, and I am unsure about the client's ability to pay close attention to his or her own needs, wants, and boundaries, I may add, "Take a moment and make sure that's OK with you."

Joe summarized:

I think that touch well-timed, as with Gestalt body therapy, can speed therapy. There are times when touch has helped me realize what was going on at the time. I think talk has been overall most important, but a combination of the two speeds things up.

Minimal or No Use of Touch in Therapy

Extreme Sexual, Physical, and/or Emotional Abuse and/or Neglect

Although it has been my experience that survivors of extreme abuse and/or neglect are often those who benefit the most from touch in therapy, the opposite can also be true. Lacy and Tom are cases in point.

Client 6: Lacy. It may be that a person's ability to touch and be touched corresponds roughly to that person's psychological and emotional tolerance for closeness. Lacy wrote in her questionnaire, "It takes me time and extreme comfort and safety to allow touch. I allow people I trust/love to touch me and enjoy touching them." Lacy did not ever reach that level of trust or love with me or with the other members of the women's therapy group she was in for 2 years.

Lacy was sexually abused by her uncle when she was between the ages of 4 and 12. This childhood experience set up in her an extreme distaste for and distrust of touch outside the context of well-established relationships proven "safe" over time. Although Lacy received "warm, loving, comfortable touch" from her mother as a child, the mother did nothing to stop the sexual abuse when Lacy told her about it as a very young child. This betrayal was more devastating to her than the abuse itself.

Lacy was just as explicit in writing about her experience of touch in psychotherapy as she was in the actual context of the group: "It is voluntary, for the most part, and generally requested by individual group members. I find it extremely uncomfortable and don't want to participate or be touched." The words "for the most part" stand out for me. This implies that there may have been some touch that she perceived as not being totally voluntary. Perhaps this motivated her initially to leave as soon as the session was over, when others were hugging one another good-bye, as well as to use other nonverbal distancing mechanisms, such as making limited eye contact. Once Lacy had established her feelings about touch with the group, she was able to linger for good-byes without fear of someone's invading her physically. She also seemed to be more present and made more contact with others within therapy sessions after she had been clear about not wanting to participate in any therapeutic touch in the group.

However, she withdrew into her own world whenever another group member did deep feeling release work that involved touch. When I noticed that this type of work scared her, I invited to her to talk about her fears. I also told her to feel free to leave the group during such work and rejoin us later. Although she never exercised this option, it made her feel more comfortable to know she did not have to be "stuck" in this scary situation, as she felt "stuck" as a child at the hands of her abuser.

Lacy was toward the end of her stay in the group when she completed the questionnaire on touch in therapy. To the question "What do you want your therapist to know about you and touch in psychotherapy?", she responded, "That I don't want to be touched—*yet* [emphasis added]. I would like to be flexible about this, but at the moment it is out of the question."

Although Lacy expressed a mild interest in being "flexible" about touch, she did not choose to explore this possibility before she decided to leave the group. Upon leaving, she said that the group never had felt quite comfortable or safe to her. She was unable to answer the group members' or my inquiries about what might have made the group safer for her. She did write in the questionnaire, however, that touch interfered with her process in therapy by making her "feel inadequate at times."

In retrospect, I believe Lacy is an example of a client who might have fared better in a group in which touch was not used at all. Various touch modalities used in this long-term group, where trust among most members was already well established when Lacy became a member, was enough to make her feel inadequate and prevent her from feeling safe enough to establish the verbal contact over time that would have given her more trust and comfort in the group.

Client 9: Tom. Although Tom wanted more than anything else to have a relationship with a woman, he had been disappointed in love several times. He usually began relationships with beautifully handwritten, creative letters, but found himself unable to sustain close contact in person.

Tom is an extreme introvert who takes extraordinary measures to avoid being around many people at once, such as grocery shopping at 3:00 in the morning. He derives no pleasure from much that is ordinary or sublime—not from eating a good meal, not from a beautiful spring day, not from an orange sunset behind silver-lined clouds. The few interests that engage him—reading biographies of people whose lives in some way resemble his own, listening to music, and watching rented movies on his VCR—do not require him to venture outside his home, where he feels the most content and the least fearful.

Tom has little contact with his siblings, although his mother and favorite sister live within 100 miles. Although he is "underemployed" from an intellectual standpoint (he is very bright), his job is well suited to him emotionally and interpersonally. The job is routine, predictable, and highly structured; allows him to function autonomously; and requires him to interact only sparingly with other people. If I have painted a picture of sparseness, I have given you an accurate view of the landscape of Tom's life. But this is only the external view. Internally, Tom feels unworthy, unacceptable, angry, and misunderstood. He compares himself to the monster in *Frankenstein,* who is basically good and decent, but becomes angry and destructive because he feels misunderstood. He also identifies with the Phantom in *The Phantom of the Opera,* who is shunned because of his external flaws, rather than appreciated for his musical talent and loving heart.

I have described Tom rather extensively because his succinct responses to the questions on the touch questionnaire reflected only the sparsity and not the intricacy of his personality. About the history of touch in his family of origin, Tom wrote only this: "I was seldom touched. I was ridiculed by my father for being touched by the women in my family (mother, aunts, cousins, grandmothers). As a result, I didn't like to be touched." What Tom did not write, because it was not related to touch per se, is that his father also teased him unmercifully as a prepubescent child when he had girls as friends. He also criticized Tom harshly for any way in which he did not conform to what he thought a proper boy should be. He insisted on straight-A performance in school (no A-minuses were allowed), and demanded that Tom quit the band and play football. Neither parent supported Tom in pursuing his extraordinary artistic talent; his father deemed it "sissy," and his mother told him that he could never make a living "that way."

Fear of ridicule and external demands have thus been the central motivating factors in Tom's adaptation to life. He can hardly bear even now to have people know anything about him—even his age or where he lives—for fear of giving them an inroad into his life, and thus the ability to hurt him.

About his current experience of touch in psychotherapy, Tom said tersely, "My therapist does not touch me." About his personal experience of being touched in therapy, he noted, "Initially, my therapist gave me a hug after session. Not any more." He answered "Nothing" to the question "What do you want your therapist to know about you and touch in psychotherapy?" He stated that he gives his therapist no cues about touch because he is "indifferent" to it. Furthermore, in one or two-word phrases, Tom wrote that touch has neither interfered with nor facilitated nor contributed to his therapy. Tom described helpful touch as "being touched if I wanted it" and unhelpful touch as "being touched when I don't want it."

I offered Tom a brief hug at the end of a few sessions toward the beginning of therapy to "test the waters," so to speak—that is, to see if he could respond at all to human touch. Although he hugged me back in a mechanical sort of way, his body was rigid and unresponsive; this conveyed to me a nonverbal "don't touch" message. A danger of touching and then withdrawing touch is that a client may feel that he or she has done something wrong, or that the therapist finds him or her untouchable and therefore unlovable. Tom told me, however, that my hugging him did not "bother" him, and that my not hugging him had no impact except that he no longer had to attend to it.

Although I occasionally *do* touch Tom lightly on the knee during a session or on his shoulder as he leaves my office to convey my genuine affection for him, he did not acknowledge this in the questionnaire. I continue to hope that he may conclude that if I find him touchable, someone else might also find him touchable and lovable; even more importantly, he may learn a bit about loving himself. This has not yet happened for Tom. He tells me that when people (mostly women) touch him on the arm during conversation, he is more aware of the touch itself than of the contact they intend to make. He still imagines his father ridiculing him for touching, as he did when Tom was a child.

Since an occasional touch does not "bother" Tom, or alienate him from therapy, I will continue to touch him lightly from time to time to draw attention to his issues surrounding touch and to encourage further awareness and "working through" of his unfinished business with his father.

I have not touched Tom more extensively (1) because he has given no indication that he wants to be touched; and (2) because he does not yet have the adequate ego strength or environmental support to cope with the powerful feelings of rage, terror, and grief that could be unleashed with therapeutic touch techniques. Tom's therapy is important to him—he hasn't missed a session in 7 years. It provides him a safe place to "be known" without fear of recrimination; it helps him be aware of and express his feelings; and it helps him maintain his current level of functioning. But I feel that most touch techniques are counterindicated for him at this time.

Unmet Dependency Needs during Childhood, with Little Current Environmental Support

I received no questionnaires from anyone who fit well into the last category. But I believe that this is a type of client well worth discussing at least briefly, based on my clinical experience. Such a client is not a good candidate for touch.

This would be a client whose dependency needs went unmet during childhood, and who has insufficient ego strength or adult functioning to allow differentiation between a pervasive wish to be reparented passively and a wish for *some* reparenting. In Gestalt therapy, we consider movement toward psychological health as movement from environmental support to self-support. Self-support includes a balance between the ability to take care of oneself and the ability to reach out into the environment to get one's needs met.

A passive, dependent client believes that the therapist alone will be the savior and will provide *all* the nurturance, love, and support the client did not receive as a child. There may be in such clients a sense of entitlement that says, "I didn't get what I needed as a child, and you, the therapist, *should* provide it for me." Such clients take little responsibility either for reaching into themselves for self-support, or for reaching out into the environment outside the therapy office for support from other people, situations, or resources. I do not believe it is wise to touch such clients until a more cognitive approach has been successful in building up the adult functioning the clients need to be self-empowered. Holding or body work in a regressed state with such a client can easily be misinterpreted by the client as meaning that the therapist will take on the role of the longed-for substitute parent.

SUMMARY AND CONCLUSIONS

The goal in Gestalt therapy is to help clients achieve satisfaction in living by moving smoothly and fully through the phases of the contact–withdrawal cycle. This involves both awareness of feelings and needs, and the expression of those feelings and needs in action and interaction.

The body often reveals awarenesses not yet available to cognition or verbalization (e.g., in a chronically furrowed brow or a foot in constant motion). By noticing such nonverbal cues and bringing them to our clients' attention, we therapists can speed the acquisition of awareness. Then, with well-timed and well-positioned touch, we can often facilitate the expression of action or interaction that is retroflected in the body. If we listen only to clients' words, we will miss, and they will miss, some of the most profound realities of their existence.

Touch versus Talk

If we only talk and refuse to touch, we may miss, and clients may miss, an opportunity to find an inroad to the unexpressed feelings that are blocking their ability to live and love fully. Touch is an infant's first and most intimate human contact. Touch may sometimes reach all the way to a soul that is deaf to words alone.

Promotion of Dialogue and Learning from Mistakes

Clients need to feel free to express their wishes about being or not being touched. They also need to be invited to discuss their experiences of touch, both positive and negative. Finally, they need to know that the therapist will be nondefensive if they reveal that touch has in any way been problematic for them.

Movement from Environmental Support to Self-Support

Fritz Perls (1969) is well known for his view that "maturing is the transcendence from environmental support to self-support" (p. 30). I do not, as a Gestalt therapist of feminist persuasion, agree with Perls's extreme philosophy of self-reliance; rather, I promote a balance of independence and interrelatedness. However, I do believe that touch used in the context of therapy needs to support the maturation of clients by assisting them over time in relying less and less on their therapists, and more and more on their own resources outside therapy. Any touch that does not seem to serve in the direction of this goal needs to be evaluated and modified.

Individualizing Use of Touch

There was and is a wide range in the extent and modalities of touch used in therapy with the clients discussed above, as well as with the 25 clients whose questionnaires I have not reviewed in this chapter. Several criteria are useful in determining whether or how to use touch as a therapeutic tool. These include a client's childhood history of touch; verbal and nonverbal cues from the client; the developmental level at which the client is working (preverbal, nonverbal, verbal); the client's current personal and professional functioning; his or her degree of dependence on the therapist; and the client's availability and use of support systems outside of therapy. No one criterion can be used alone to make such determinations.

Neither can we rely solely on clusters of traits, although certain configurations may be quite useful in helping a therapist make clinical judgments about the use of touch. For example, Lacy resembled, on most dimensions, many other sexual abuse survivors with whom I gradually introduced touch and eventually used it extensively. However, I did not even broach the subject of touch in therapy with Lacy, because I judged it to be therapeutically crucial to respect her negative feelings about touch, and also because the therapeutic alliance was not strong enough for me to feel that suggesting touch was a possibility.

Just as I have not yet met one client who fits precisely and wholly into one DSM-IV diagnostic category, I have not met one client who responds precisely like any other to the use of therapeutic touch. The total Gestalt and the special uniqueness of each client must be taken into consideration. Combined with solid training, a commitment to ongoing learning, a large quantity of humility, skilled clinical judgment, and finely tuned intuition, touch in the context of overall good psychotherapy can be immensely effective.

NOTES

1. All names and other demographic data, as well as various other details, have been changed to obscure the identity of clients. All clients have read the sections referring to them and have given permission to use the text as written.
2. At the Gestalt Institute of Georgia, we teach in part by demonstrating Gestalt work with trainees as "clients," and we integrate the attention to

body movement and expression that is inherent in traditional Gestalt therapy with hands-on approaches borrowed from other therapeutic approaches. (See Smith, 1985.)

3. Smith (1985) notes:

> In both presentification and regression the patient creates a here-and-now experience, feeling the emotion of the historical incident as the incident is remembered and relived. In the case of regression, the patient is encouraged to "go back" to the age at which the incident in question occurred, feeling and being as much as possible that age. (With presentification, on the other hand, the patient brings the past forward in time so that the old incident is relived with the patient being as he or she is now.) Regression is called for when the task is to let the patient gain awareness by re-experiencing how it was to be a child in the historical situation. . . . Regression is also appropriate when the task is to give the patient the experience of getting a childhood need met, which in literal childhood was not met adequately. (p. 56)

REFERENCES

Kepner, J. I. (1987). *Body process.* New York: Gardner Press.

Miller, A. (1981). *The drama of the gifted child.* New York: Basic Books.

Perls, F. S. (1969). *Gestalt therapy verbatim.* Moab, UT: Real People Press.

Polster, E., & Polster, M. (1974). *Gestalt therapy integrated.* New York: Vintage Books.

Schreiber, F. R. (1973). *Sybil.* New York: Warner.

Smith, E. W. L. (1985). *The body in psychotherapy.* Jefferson, NC: McFarland.

13

TOUCH AND CLIENTS WHO HAVE BEEN SEXUALLY ABUSED

Suzann Smith Lawry

It is unequivocal that touch is a natural and essential part of human development and communication. One need only recall Harlow's often-cited monkeys (Harlow & Zimmerman, 1959), or the numerous studies showing babies failing to thrive in environments with little or no touch for testimony of this truth (Hainline & Krinsky-McHale, 1994). Since touch is a natural and normal feature of human relationships, it follows that the *absence* of touch in human encounters is unavoidably a communication. It is our ethical and professional responsibility as therapists to be aware of our communications to our clients both verbally and nonverbally. Thus, we must examine closely the ramifications of our positions on touch in psychotherapy, to avoid naively allowing its absence *or* presence to affect the therapeutic process haphazardly.

One population deserving particular consideration in this regard consists of adult survivors of childhood sexual abuse. For this group, touch has often been an integral part of their early trauma, and consequently touch may have a variety of idiosyncratic meanings. Moreover, because of some of the specific sequelae with which many survivors struggle, the assessment of whether to utilize touch can be extremely complicated. And finally, it has been shown that clients with a history of sexual abuse have a higher likelihood of being revictimized sexually *by their therapists* (Gutheil, 1991). Consequently, particular attention to the use of touch interventions with this population is warranted.

Due to these complexities, it could be argued that therapeutic touch with survivors of sexual abuse is contraindicated at all times. Given the myriad of ways in which touch, even well-intentioned touch, can be subjectively experienced as harmful, abstaining from using touch interventions with survivors is certainly a viable option. Moreover, it may very well be the position of choice for beginning therapists, for therapists who employ short-term treatment modalities, for therapists who are uncomfortable with touch themselves, and for all others as a "default" position when there is *any* question as to the therapeutic benefit and appropriateness of touch.

If a clinician has adopted the position of abstinence from touch in therapy, it is important to discuss the rationale for this overtly with the survivor. In this way, the absence of touch is not left to communicate messages that the clinician does not intend to send (e.g., "You are too dirty to touch," or "If I touch you, I will lose my self-control"). This discussion should also make it clear that the therapeutic relationship will be an intimate but not a sexual one, and that the therapist is ultimately responsible for maintaining that boundary. This is not only good therapeutic practice (Cole & Schaefer, 1986); it is imperative with survivors of sexual abuse.

If clinicians are not beginning therapists, are not working within a short-term model of treatment, and are otherwise comfortable with the use of touch, then the following guidelines are offered for the decision-making process of whether to utilize touch with particular sexual abuse survivors. As with any therapeutic intervention, its use should be evaluated for each client *individually*. Furthermore, nothing, including these guidelines, can replace careful and honest self-scrutiny, peer review, and adequate supervision. However, the present guidelines can facilitate these processes in work with survivors of childhood sexual abuse.

QUESTIONS TO ASK ABOUT YOURSELF

"How Do I Feel about Touch Personally?"

If touch is uncomfortable for you, it doesn't matter whether or not your theoretical position incorporates touching interventions; you will not be able to utilize touch effectively until your issues are resolved. Relatedly, if you are uneasy about touching a particular client for reasons known or unknown, heed your internal warning. Your comfort with touch is a therapeutic prerequisite for considering using it with any clients, sexual abuse survivors included. However, if you value the use of touch in psychotherapy and you are unable to touch a client comfortably (for whatever reasons), you may consider having him or her work with a massage therapist, a group therapist, or the client's partner, in conjunction with therapy. For example, if a client feels that his or her body is unable to receive any comfort or pleasure from physical contact, a referral to a massage therapist or sensate focus exercises with the client's partner may be beneficial. It is, of course, important for such a third party to be respectful of the client's pace and not to be abusive in any way.

"Am I Attracted Sexually to This Client?"

If you are sexually attracted to *any* client, it is not the time to use touch therapeutically. Moreover, given the increased risk for survivors to be reabused by their therapists, avoiding using touch interventions at such times is even more critical for this population. However, at such times it is wise to secure good supervision and attend to your own intimacy and sexual needs. If the attraction is unresolvable, then a referral is warranted. Acting out the attraction is never justifiable.

The negative effects on clients of having sex with their therapists have clearly been identified: increased depression, suicidality, feelings of betrayal, difficulty in trusting others, guilt, and self-loathing (Brown, 1988; Feldman-Summers & Jones, 1984; Sonne, Meyer, Borys, & Marshall, 1985; Sonne & Pope, 1991). The similarity of these symptoms to sexual abuse sequelae is obvious. Thus, when a therapist recapitulates the original trauma by violating a sexual boundary again, this is inexcusable ethically, therapeutically, and theoretically.

Abel, Lawry, and Osborn (1994) factor-analyzed items that were endorsed by over 150 male professionals as having contributed to their self-admitted sexual misconduct. This analysis yielded four types of offenders. The first was the offender who felt he was uniquely able to meet his clients' needs. The second was the offender who was particularly emotionally and/or physically needy. The third type was the offender who felt there was little chance of getting caught. And, finally, the fourth was a more passive type of offender who attributed the sexual misconduct to his attractive and seductive victims.

The relevance of the Abel et al. research to the present discussion is that therapists may benefit by paying close attention to early signs of each of these four dynamics to avoid sexual misconduct with their clients. With regard to the first dynamic, ask yourself if there is a "therapist-as-savior" dynamic operating. Do you feel that you are the one and only person to provide for the emotional and/or physical needs of your client(s)? Do you consistently go beyond your normal practice in terms of meeting a particular client's needs and emergencies? If so, this may be indicative of a problem. In this scenario, early preventive action should include reestablishing your normal therapeutic boundaries and facilitating the development of your client's support systems. In addition, exploring such grandiosity in personal therapy and/or professional supervision is advisable.

Second, are you particularly sexually or emotionally needy right now? We all vary in our emotional and physical needs across therapy; however, if touching your client feels healing for *you*, or the impulse to touch comes from *your* own sexual or emotional needs, then immediate steps should be taken to stop, address your needs outside the therapeutic setting, and (of course) secure adequate supervision. Again, you may not be aware that you are touching a client because of your own needs. Thus, paying attention to early signs of this dynamic may prevent you from acting it out. Early warning signs include rapid increases in your self-disclosures or touching only one type of client, for example, only attractive clients. Certainly, if you have recently experienced significant losses in your personal life, it would be an important time to exert care in monitoring your own need gratification.

Third, are you taking steps to keep your touching of your client(s) a secret? This can be as overt as telling a client not to tell others because "others wouldn't understand," or as subtle as avoiding discussing your touching interventions in peer and/or formal supervision. The frequency of the latter prompted Wilson (1982) to state, "It may be that the touch taboo is not deterring many therapists from using touch, but is strong enough to keep them from admitting it to one another" (p. 66). This state of affairs is a fertile ground for unsound decisions and for the recapitulation of keeping secrets with abuse survivors.

Finally, have you avoided working through individually and in supervision how you would respond to an overt or covert solicitation for sexual contact by a client? Some sexual abuse survivors acquired a small measure of control by initiating the sexual contact with their perpetrator(s). In addition, some survivors have no schemas for intimate relationships or nurturance other than sexual ones. These are a few of the many reasons why a survivor may, at some point in therapy, try to sexualize the therapeutic relationship. Thus, avoiding discussion of what you would do at such a juncture, and failing to develop a clear therapeutic guideline, are naive if you are working with this population. (For further discussion of what to do if a client seeks sexual gratification from you, see below.)

If you have answered yes to any of these four questions, it doesn't necessarily mean that you are committing sexual misconduct. However, since these four dynamics have been identified by offenders who *have* engaged in sexual misconduct, close attention should be given to these issues both individually and in supervision. The use of therapeutic touch should be either delayed until they are resolved, or avoiding altogether.

QUESTIONS TO ASK ABOUT YOUR CLIENT

"What Client Need Is Being Met by Touch, and Is Touch the Only Way of Meeting That Need?"

Certainly some of the therapeutic benefits of touch that have been identified in the literature—such as increasing self-disclosure, providing containment, communicating empathy, increasing the client's interpersonal risk taking, and enhancing the therapeutic alliance (Dies & Greenberg, 1976; Horton, Clance, Sterk-Elifson, & Emshoff, 1995; Wilson, 1982)—may be achieved through other, nonphysical therapeutic interventions. Given the complexities of using touch with sexual abuse survivors, when another method or technique is equally effective, it should be used.

However, it does appear that there are times when touch can provide unique therapeutic communications, such as, "You are touchable," "Touch can feel safe and nurturing," or "You can say no or yes to touch." These communications are particularly important to a survivor of sexual trauma. Finkelhor (1986), in a somewhat simplistic but clinically useful model, outlined four traumagenic factors that can exacerbate and/or mitigate a survivor's symptomatology following sexual trauma. The first is stigmatization; that is, the client feels different from everyone and uniquely "bad." The client's experiencing that he or she is touchable can be an antidote to stigmatization. In addition, experiencing touch that is safe and nurturing can directly counter the second traumagenic factor, betrayal (and the resulting difficulty in trusting others). Safe and nurturing touch is also relevant to the third traumagenic factor, sexualization (i.e., the belief that all touch is sexual, which can result in either avoidance of all touch or overly sexualized behavior). And finally, being able to say yes or no to touch provides the client with an experience that can mitigate the fourth traumagenic factor, powerlessness (especially with regard to the client's own body). These and other benefits of touch are beginning to be empirically supported. In a study of touch in psychotherapy, a subsample of survivors (who were either sexually abused or both physically and sexually abused) reported that touching interventions in their therapy "repaired self-esteem, trust, and a sense of their own power or agency, especially in setting limits and asking for what they needed" (Horton et al., 1995, p. 452; see also Chapter 9 of this volume, p. 132).

"Does My Client Have Sufficient Ego Strength?"

A client's ego strength can be difficult to assess. One of its hallmarks is a history of being able to process interpersonal material with you when needed. For example, has this client been able to disagree with you, inquire about process, and/or check out faulty assumptions? A related but distinct issue is whether your client has been able to set limits with powerful figures in his or her life. A common axiom in training for work with sexual abuse survivors is "Before you touch, ask." However, while this may certainly be easier than taking the steps outlined in these guidelines, it is insufficient. It is insufficient because it denies the power differential inherent in therapeutic relationships. You often have to go no further than a survivor's own history to see evidence of this truth. Frequently, survivors of incest will report that they "agreed" to their abuse. Although you may clearly see the power differential and discount such "agreements," you may not see the same dynamic in "asking" clients for permission to touch them when they may not have the ego strength to refuse. While asking or at the least announcing your intentions is certainly preferable over touching im-pulsively without warning, it does not take the place of carefully evaluating yourself and your client in each of these areas.

Another complicating factor in the use of touch with sexual abuse survivors is the possibility of multiple ego states, which may each have its own level of ego strength. This makes assessment more complex, but all the more important. For example, a client's adult "professional self" may be able to assert, process, and negotiate power easily, but if a "child self" is receiving the touch, it is the child self's ego strength that needs to be understood. When you are working with a client with varying ego states, the most conservative position would be to aim your work toward the lowest common denominator—that is, to address interventions, including touch, to the least devel-oped ego state. The exception to this would be a case in which, through a long history of therapy, you and your client have developed clear and unerring communication when ego states are shifting and when more than one ego state is present. In this way, you can target an intervention toward one ego state and be certain that the same ego state receives it.

"What Level of Dissociation/Depersonalization Is the Client Currently Experiencing?"

If your client is having unpredictable episodes of depersonalization, flashbacks, or body memories, this is not the time to utilize therapeutic touch. During these types of experiences, there is no way to assess the potential impact of your touch or to guard against its being experienced traumatically. It should be underscored that during such times, the impulse can be quite strong to touch a client to get him or her to "come out of it," and yet such an act can all too frequently recapitulate the original trauma. Your well-intentioned pat on the shoulder, for instance, can be perceived as hands holding the client down. At such times, intermediate steps are needed before touch is used. For example, if you want a dissociative client to reconnect to the here-and-now experience of being safe in your office, slowly helping the client look at you can be quite effective. The connection that occurs when the eyes meet often interrupts dissociation and other altered states. This has been proposed to be related to the incompatibility between shame and connection (R. Simmermon, personal communication, July 12, 1996).

"Is My Client Seeking Sexual Gratification from Me?"

If a client is seeking sexual gratification from you, then it can be more difficult for the client to receive touch in the nonerotic manner that you intend. If you knowingly touch a client to stimulate or gratify his or her sexual needs, you have crossed the boundary into sexual misconduct (see above). Of course, in any therapeutic relationship, and particularly in one with a survivor of childhood sexual abuse, it is quite common for the client to be attracted to the therapist. If this is the case, but you have discussed the attraction openly and with clear boundaries, you are in a much better position to utilize touch. If the attraction has been left unprocessed, touch can easily be misconstrued. In processing clients' attractions to you it is important to explore it in the same ways you would explore any transference. In terms of process, a client's sexual solicitation may have a variety of functions. Thus, it is important to note both the interpersonal process—for example, "Your proposition sure made us stop talking about the abuse"—as well as exploring and interpreting the intrapsychic process—for example, "So it feels like if we had sex you'd feel more in control." And then, of course, setting respectful and unyielding boundaries—for example, "I want you to know, however strong your feelings are, I value you and our work together too much to allow it to ever become a sexual relationship."

"Is the Relationship Developed and Balanced Enough to Withstand the Potential Intensity of Touch?"

As has been suggested elsewhere (Wilson, 1982), it is not appropriate to use touch during the introductory phase of treatment, when the therapeutic alliance is being built. This is due to the enormous power differential between a "stranger professional" and a "seeker of help." In addition, it is impossible so early in the relationship to make an adequate assessment of the client's readiness for touch. Thus, in early sessions with any client and particularly with a sexual abuse survivor, touch is contraindicated. This is true even if a survivor "opens up" immediately; such behavior is more likely to be reflective of the individual's dynamics than of any miraculous development of therapeutic alliance in the first session.

A related power differential issue is raised by Alyn (1988), who has emphasized how the oppression of women in Western society is reflected in the high frequency of females' being casually touched in nonintimate relationships, compared to their male counterparts. This state of affairs, according to Alyn, makes male therapists' touching female clients contraindicated at all times. However, Horton et al. (1995) found that the gender composition of the dyad did not determine whether or not touch was experienced positively. Although prohibiting male therapists from touching female clients may be premature, the oppression of women underscores the need for male therapists to give particular attention to power dynamics and to the development of trust before utilizing touch interventions with female clients. In addition, it emphasizes the need for male therapists to be particularly aware of any nondeliberate touching within the therapeutic arena. Such cautions are also necessary (albeit perhaps to a lesser extent) for female therapists, because the role of therapist *alone,* brings a power differential into the therapeutic setting regardless of the gender composition of the therapeutic dyad. As a therapist, regardless of your gender, you should be constantly aware of this differential in order to utilize your power and your touch interventions effectively.

A related question is whether the relationship is strong enough to tolerate processing any therapeutic miscalculations regarding touch as "grist for the mill." There will always be times when therapeutic interventions are ill timed, misunderstood, or even misused. Touch is no different in this regard. No therapist will be perfect in the legitimate application of this technique. If you commit such honest errors, they should be owned and processed. The difference between this and other therapeutic "grist" is that the affect triggered by errors in touch may be greater and the injunctions not to discuss them may be stronger.

Remember, injunctions to be silent are particularly potent for survivors of sexual abuse. It is important to know that the relationship can tolerate a worst-case scenario before you embark upon the use of touch.

CONCLUSION

In conclusion, if I can be afforded a moment of self-disclosure, the process of writing this chapter was quite disturbing. It was disturbing because of my fear that a therapist, through either inexperience or malevolence, might use my words to justify the use of exploitative touch with sexual abuse survivors. My knowledge of the frequency in which survivors are revictimized, coupled with my witnessing their resulting pain, fueled this fear. However, my also having witnessed the power and ancient authority of touch fueled a deeper knowing that *not* writing this chapter would have been a betrayal to those whose stories, hands, and hearts I have held. In closing, the following blessing is offered in the hope that this chapter's message is received as it was intended.

> May you be at peace
> may your heart remain open
> may you awaken to the light of your own true nature
> may you be healed
> may you be a source of healing for all beings.
> (Borysenko & Slav-Borysenko, 1994, p. 128)

REFERENCES

Abel, G., Lawry, S. S., & Osborn, C. (1994). *Categorization of individuals involved in professional sexual misconduct: Implications for treatment.* Paper presented at the 13th Annual Research and Treatment Conference of the Association for the Treatment of Sexual Abusers, San Francisco.

Alyn, J. (1988). The politics of touch in therapy: A response to Willison and Masson. *Journal of Counseling and Development, 66,* 432–433.

Borysenko, J., & Slav-Borysenko, M. (1994). *The power of the mind to heal: Renewing body, mind, and spirit.* Carlsbad, CA: Hay House.

Brown, L. (1988). Harmful effects of post-termination sexual and romantic relationships with former clients. *Psychotherapy, 25,* 249–255.

Cole, E., & Schaefer, S. (1986). Boundaries of sex and intimacy between client and counselor. *Journal of Counseling and Development, 64,* 341–344.

Dies, R., & Greenberg, B. (1976). Sex effects of physical contact in an encounter group context. *Journal of Consulting and Clinical Psychology, 44*(3), 400–405.

Feldman-Summers, S., & Jones, G. (1984). Psychological impacts of sexual contact between therapists or other health care professionals and their clients. *Journal of Consulting and Clinical Psychology, 52,* 1054–1061.

Finkelhor, D. (1986). *A sourcebook on child sexual abuse.* Beverly Hills, CA: Sage.

Gutheil, T. (1991). Patients involved in sexual misconduct with therapists: Is a victim profile possible? *Psychiatric Annals, 21*(11), 661–667.

Harlow, H., & Zimmerman, R. (1959). Affectional responses in the infant monkey. *Science, 130,* 421–432.

Hainline, L., & Krinsky-McHale, S. (1994). Hurting while helping?: The paradox of the neonatal intensive care unit. *Children's Environments, 11*(2), 105–122.

Horton, J., Clance, P., Sterk-Elifson, C., & Emshoff, J. (1995). Touch in psychotherapy: A survey of patients' experiences. *Psychotherapy, 32*(3), 443–457.

Kardener, S., Fuller, M., & Mensh, I. (1976). Characteristics of "erotic" practitioners. *American Journal of Orthopsychiatry, 133*(11), 1324–1325.

Sonne, J., Meyer, C., Borys, D., & Marshall, V. (1985). Clients' reactions to sexual intimacy in therapy. *American Journal of Orthopsychiatry, 55*(2), 183–189.

Sonne, J., & Pope, K. (1991). Treating victims of therapist–patient sexual involvement. *Psychotherapy, 28,* 174–187.

Willison, B., & Masson, R. (1986). The role of touch in therapy: An adjunct to communications. *Journal of Counseling and Development, 65,* 497–500.

Wilson, J. (1982). The value of touch in psychotherapy. *American Journal of Orthopsychiatry, 52*(1), 65–72.

14

THE IMPACT OF PHYSICAL TOUCH ON PROFESSIONAL DEVELOPMENT

David Mandelbaum

A couple of years ago, I was pursuing my search for malpractice insurance coverage that would be both comprehensive and cost-effective. I had received an advertisement from a company promising comparable coverage to the policy sponsored by the American Psychological Association (APA), but at a much less costly premium. When I received the application, the basic coverage was in fact offered at a significantly reduced premium. However, the application form also included a series of questions about whether I engaged in such areas of practice as sex therapy, body work, and hypnosis. Affirmative answers to any of these questions increased the premiums significantly. Since I do incorporate body work in my practice, and occasionally hypnosis as well, not only was I not going to save any money with this company; my premiums would have been even higher. What was clear was that a therapist who did body work with (in other words, physically touched) a client was considered a much higher risk to insure than one who practiced in more traditional ways. Clearly, this company had concluded that therapists who chose to touch clients had a greater likelihood of being sued than others.

I was aware of both understanding the insurance company's position and feeling somewhat sad. My experience with body work as a client has never brought me close to being treated in an unethical manner. Nor in my work as a practicing therapist have I gone beyond the bounds of ethical treatment with my clients. For me, the experience of touch has been powerful. Indeed, in this era emphasizing shorter-term therapy, I've seen the effects of touch facilitate the working through of material that, in more traditional approaches, would have taken far longer to accomplish. What can be concluded, however, is that the use of touch in the therapeutic process is considered risky and controversial. How an awareness of this risk and controversy has had an impact on me in my practice is one of the areas I discuss in this chapter.

MY TRAINING AS A PSYCHOTHERAPIST

After receiving my master's degree in school psychology and completing my internship, I decided to transfer to the Division of Individual and Family Studies in the College of Human Development at Penn State University. In 1972, I began studying with Bernard and Louise Guerney, who were professors in the College of Human Development. They had developed a series of therapeutic interventions based upon an educational model. That spring, a number of graduate students in the department, including me, had a brief experience with Gestalt therapy. The experience was so exciting and so unlike anything that I had been exposed to up to that point that a group of us contacted a professor in the psychology department whom we had heard was a Gestalt therapist and arranged a weekend Gestalt experience. That time of my life was a painful one, because I had separated about 2 months earlier from my first wife and my then 8-month-old son. During the weekend I volunteered to work, and the facilitator had me engage in dialogue with my son about the separation and my leaving him. I experienced a rush of intense grief. While I was sobbing, the facilitator came over and asked me to turn over on my back. He placed his hand on my chest and gently rubbed the area over my heart. I was astounded at how comforting that felt. When I completed the experience, I was surprised at my relief. I felt more resolution in that 20-minute piece of work than I had experienced in the 2 months of therapy I had been in up to that point. Although the weekend wasn't set up to be a training experience per se, it was my first in-depth exposure to Gestalt therapy, and it affected me profoundly. I was in a dilemma, however: This approach was significantly different from the relationship enhancement (RE) approach developed by the Guerneys. Although RE was a powerful educational tool, it was essentially cognitive in nature because of its skill training and homework requirements. As a result, it didn't permit the recognition and working through of powerful complexes that might interfere with the development of meaningful and satisfying relationships. Gestalt, on the other hand, tapped into deep and heartfelt emotions in a relatively brief period of time and provided a structure for that working through. Since I was a young graduate student, I hadn't yet learned the simple resolution to the dilemma: Both were viable approaches. Perhaps even more importantly, I began, even then, to think of ways in which certain Gestalt therapy skills (deepening awareness, dialoguing) might be taught to clients for use on their own.

I continued to feel very positive about the Gestalt approach. But over the next several years, I began to hear rumors about Fritz Perls's blind spots in his work with clients. I also had an unsettling experience involving a colleague at Elmira College (where I was now directing the counseling center). The colleague, in my opinion, had caused some relatively minor damage to students by allowing seniors who had participated in a Gestalt retreat to conduct unsupervised Gestalt therapy with younger students. This left the practitioners extremely uneasy, and they had come to me with their concerns. I was able to confront the colleague, and the practice quickly ceased. As a result, though I was still impressed with the power of the approach, I had become somewhat less naive about the fact that this approach, like any other, could be misapplied. Yet I was so impressed with a Gestalt seminar I attended that I decided to enroll in a year-long training experience in existential–Gestalt therapy, beginning in January 1981. Since this experience was so literally life-changing, I would like to describe it in some detail.

The experience of touch was a primary factor in the training process and was highly significant. I experienced it in many ways during the Gestalt training. First, it was built into several facets of the training itself. It was there that I received my first exposure to Edward Smith's (1979) writing on the "contact–withdrawal cycle" and its relevance to working with the body in psychotherapy, of which I will say much more later. Second, the trainer, a gifted Gestalt therapist, demonstrated the use of ethical touch in the therapeutic process, and I was privileged to be a witness to some transforming experiences. Third, over a period of a year of intense work, the group members developed a cohesiveness that allowed for playful physical interaction with each other. However, I cannot say that the training was valuable for every participant; it wasn't. In many ways, this first training group was similar to the life phase of adolescence. Participants were exposed to new skills and experimented with stretching their boundaries, as often occurs during adolescence. In the process of stretching these boundaries through touch, there was, on occasion, some unconscious acting out. Specifically, a couple of group members initiated relationships with others. Although these relationships were not kept secret, my sense was that not all parties involved were always fully aware of the possible impact on the group. As a result, much time was spent in the group processing the impact of these relationships, and this took time away from the training. And, like many adolescents, a few group members experienced some pain as a result. Yet, as in successful adolescence, the majority of participants learned important life (career) skills, which time and further training would help mature.

Several of the participants in this first group went on to continue more advanced training in further groups; in fact, a training group continues to this day, with a core of the original participants (myself included). We have also participated in a series of body workshops that have been among the most powerful training experiences I've received. These workshops began in 1990 and have occurred yearly since then. I've been fortunate enough to participate in all except one. They take place at a rustic lodge, and each lasts for 5 days. The majority of trainees have been seasoned licensed psychotherapists, and a few have been graduate students in psychology. The theory and practice derive from Edward Smith's book *The Body in Psychotherapy* (1985), and the underlying therapeutic principle is the "contact–withdrawal cycle" first described by Smith in 1979. I want to describe the cycle briefly, because it is the key to understanding both the nature and the power of the training experiences.

The contact–withdrawal cycle is a theoretical construct that describes the natural evolution of a need state beginning with one's awareness of a "want" and moving through a series of steps into appropriate expression of this want, leading to eventual satisfaction. In the best of all possible worlds (a supportive and accepting environment), an individual moves through these steps unhindered, with guidance regarding appropriate ways to satisfy the needs as they move into awareness. Unfortunately, most of us don't live in the best of all possible worlds; virtually all of us experience some degree of prohibition against awareness or expression, which we internalize partially or fully to prevent our need satisfaction. These prohibitions or rules against being fully aware and alive are called "toxic introjects" and are usually communicated to us by significant figures in our lives, such as parents, teachers, or representatives of churches/synagogues. These negative rules have two components: the particular content of prohibition ("Big boys don't cry," "Nice girls shouldn't get angry"), and the overt or implied threat of withdrawal of love from the significant figure. Because the threat of abandonment by this figure is so anxiety-arousing, the individual internalizes the negative message and eventually comes to believe that the negative message is true. As a result, the individual enacts a number of cognitive and physiological defenses against knowing the truth of his or her experience. These defenses include inhibited breathing to blocked awareness of the total feeling experience, and at times a retroflection (turning back upon the self) of action or interaction to prevent full expression of the want or need.

With chronic enactment of these defenses, muscular tension can develop. As an example, I worked with a woman whose presenting symptoms were chronic hip and leg spasms. At the first visit her legs were crossed, and one leg kept moving spasmodically in a kicking or thrusting motion. I encouraged her to breathe deeply, and she began recovering memories of childhood sexual abuse. She remembered being given to men by her mother for sexual satisfaction. The leg thrusts, when given full expression, were her way of trying to fend off the attacks by the men. Over time, she had retroflected the action into chronic spasms. Another example—perhaps one that is more familiar to the reader—is the experience of holding back tears. In order not to cry, a person usually engages in a diminishment of breath, a tightening of the throat muscles, and perhaps excessive swallowing. It takes great effort not to express that which is natural to express. This effort, if made repeatedly, will eventually produce chronic muscle tension in the throat and chest, which almost automatically kicks in whenever a sad experience begins to move into awareness. Over time, the body may begin to respond in this characteristic way without the cognitive awareness of the triggering event from the past or the present. The process by which a person internalizes a toxic introject also provides a way to increase awareness and undo its effects. In other words, sometimes the most efficient way to access the content of the toxic introject is to attend to the ways in which the body characteristically reacts to keep the individual from moving through the contact-withdrawal cycle. As a result of that attention, a therapist may be able to guide a client, with body work, through the contact-withdrawal cycle and into eventual completion or satisfaction.

Training in this type of work is very intense and often leads to explosions of grief, rage, and profound sadness. One cannot be a witness to such work without being deeply affected. The training also occurs in a group, which creates an almost synergistic effect, further intensifying the emotional experience of any one participant. Many of the participants have been together since 1990, and all have done significant personal work either with the workshop leader or with other members. The trust that has thus been established further facilitates and deepens the training effects. Because all participants stay together in a retreat setting, sharing meals and free time, there is more opportunity to contact each other and to allow awareness and appropriate expression to move. Finally, most of the participants are seasoned therapists with a level of experience and maturity that more readily allows for assimilation and integration.

Each day of the training begins with breakfast at 8:00. There are two work sessions, from 9:00 to noon and from 2:00 to 5:00. During these work sessions, the leader usually does a bit of lecturing and then demonstrates a particular technique with a volunteer. As the 5 days pass, participants usually have an opportunity to do some therapy with other volunteers, and to receive feedback from the leader and the rest of the group. As stated above, the work is often so intense that frequent breaks are necessary to allow individuals the time to withdraw and assimilate their experience. There is usually one formal evening session, with the rest of the evenings left for participants to attend to themselves and each other in ways that allow for movement through both individual and group contact–withdrawal cycles. Often there is a quiet evening; there is usually an evening that moves into music and dancing; and, almost always, joy and humor abound. In short, participants live the contact–withdrawal cycle in as supportive an environment as can be imagined.

I have noted that my earlier, year-long training experience in existential–Gestalt therapy resulted in some inappropriate boundary stretching, and I have likened that group to the developmental phase of adolescence. This experience is quite different, primarily due to the maturity and experience of the participants. In this training, boundaries are stretched but never violated. People are extremely clear about what is acceptable, and they exercise appropriate judgment and restraint while remaining true to the contact and withdrawal. Much affection is felt and expressed, but never inappropriately. It is a joy to experience. Being fully alive with people who maintain integrity in a safe and supportive environment is extraordinarily liberating and allows for the kind of experiential learning that cannot easily be obtained in any classroom situation.

MY PRACTICE OF PSYCHOTHERAPY

An article in the *APA Monitor* (DeAngelis & Mwakalyelye, 1995) described research demonstrating that infants who were regularly massaged and otherwise stroked were healthier and thrived better than those who hadn't received equivalent physical contact. Perhaps even more relevant, mothers who received massage were less depressed and anxious than those who received just relaxation training. I recall from my introductory psychology course that Spitz (1945) reported similar findings for orphaned infants many years ago. In addition, the appropriateness of having physical contact with a child while conducting nondirective play therapy is not often questioned. Why, then, is touch such a controversial issue in doing therapy with adults? Clearly, there are unprofessional and unethical therapists, but why throw the baby out with the bathwater?

Part of the reason, I suspect, has to do with a cultural toxic introject. I imagine the introject goes something like this: "Once you reach a certain age [say, about 18], you should be strong or tough enough to deal with most issues without needing to be held or otherwise to have physical support. If you need to have that type of support, you are weak, and if a therapist provides that support, he or she is probably acting out some sexual need that is out of his or her awareness." I believe this introject affects both clients and therapists, and it has certainly had an impact on how I incorporate touch in my practice.

In my work with individuals, I have incorporated body work and therapeutic touch, but only after certain criteria are met. First, the relationship has to be a fairly trusting one; thus, several sessions must have occurred in which a client feels safe and comfortable with me. I rarely, if ever, attempt body work in the first few sessions. Second, I never touch a client in any way without first asking for his or her permission. I almost always engage in a piece of didactic work explaining the contact–withdrawal cycle and describing how we can all develop "character armor" from repeatedly repressing components of either the awareness or expression ends of the cycle. Third, my preference is always to begin with the less intrusive techniques before I engage in the more hands-on strategies. The first strategy I employ does not involve direct touching, but is characterized by verbal instructions regarding the body. These may include suggestions to deepen the breathing, to shift the body position, or to become aware of tension in particular muscles and to relax those areas of the body. An example is a woman I worked with years ago who came into a session as tight as a drum. She sat on the couch, with her knees drawn up to her chest and her breathing very shallow and rapid. I instructed her to stretch out and deepen her breathing. As she did so, she immediately moved into rather deep sobbing and began reporting a very painful memory from childhood. Another example is any client who, when beginning to experience sadness, unconsciously tenses the muscles of the throat and chest and who inhibits the breathing.

Often, an instruction to deepen breathing and relax areas of muscular tension is sufficient to evoke the suppressed affect. If more work is required, I then opt for what Smith (1985) describes as "soft" techniques. These include light touch or placing the client's body in various postures that have specific meaning. Only if the suggestions and the "soft" techniques fail to lead to full awareness or expression will I resort to "hard" techniques, in which I employ deep pressure to release muscular tension. Finally, after any body work, I encourage the client to express all feelings and reactions that result from the work. I also encourage the client to ask any questions (both before and after the work) that may be necessary for his or her satisfaction. Throughout the work, I am always striving to be aware of whose needs are being served by the intervention. Any intervention should be in the service first of facilitating movement through the contact–withdrawal cycle, and second of providing the client with nurturing compassion expressed through physical contact.

Having said all of this, I must note that I personally find myself more comfortable doing body work in a group therapy setting. As I mentioned earlier, a group often has a synergistic effect, which allows for deeper awareness and experiencing at a faster pace than might be possible during individual work. Also, I find myself feeling more insulated from misunderstanding and misperception in a group setting. After all, there are many more corroborating observers, compared to an individual session. Currently, my partner and I are cofacilitating a men's therapy group that meets for 2 hours every other week. In addition, the participants (eight men ranging in age from 30 to 55) and facilitators attend two retreats a year that last 1½ days each; one of these occurs near the beginning of the group's meetings for the year, and one near the end. This group has been in continuous existence for 7 years, with two of the men having been in attendance from the beginning. Typically, from year to year, about half the people choose to continue and half are new members. During the first retreat we present the contact–withdrawal model, with particular emphasis placed upon the role and function of toxic introjects. During this first session, also, profound work usually occurs in which my partner and/or I use both "soft" body techniques and interventions that require more hands-on work. The men become very willing to participate by offering physical support for each other. Virtually all choose to work on some issue, and, almost without exception, deep transformational experiences occur. During the second retreat, usually 7 or 8 months after the first retreat and after 14 to 16 group sessions, the men have grown even more comfortable with each other and with the facilitators. As a result of the safety they have experienced, they often choose to work on even deeper personal issues than they were willing to explore during the first retreat. The second retreat provides closure for the year, and plans are made for the following year.

My continuing struggle both personally and professionally is to find ethical ways of incorporating touch in my practice, to feel safe as I do so, and to combat so many of the personal and cultural toxic introjects that make all our lives less alive and ultimately less fulfilling.

REFERENCES

DeAngelis, T., & Mwakalyelye, N. (1995, October 26). The power of touch helps vulnerable babies thrive. *APA Monitor,* p. 25.

Smith, E. (1979). Seven decision points. *Voices, 15*(3), 45–50.

Smith, E. (1985). *The body in psychotherapy.* Jefferson, NC: McFarland.

Spitz, R. A. (1945). An inquiry into the genesis of psychiatric conditions in early childhood. *Psychoanalytic Study of the Child, 1,* 53–74.

15

JEAN'S LEGACY

On the Use of Physical Touch in Long-Term Psychotherapy

Pamela Torraco

It is impossible to address the issue of physical touching without first examining nonphysical "touching." For all of us in the helping professions—physicians, the clergy, nurses, psychotherapists—it is our job to "touch" those who come to us, to make contact with them in a way no one else has. It is our job to provide a sense of safety and holding by using our very being. Physical touch is only one of the many avenues open to us.

For those of us who are therapists, our aim is to "touch our patients' souls"—to provide temporary but real relief from basic, early-life fear. "I am not afraid of what terrifies you so much," we must somehow communicate. "Your fear poses no danger to either of us. It is safe to expose it here, and together we will examine it." Words alone are insufficient. They address only the cerebral cortex, whereas the fear resides in the basic physiology, where it affects both autonomic functioning and idiosyncratic emotional reactions to normal, everyday events. Real contact can occur only when a therapist can "reach in and touch" a patient on such a deep level.

Two of the five senses routinely come into play in any face-to-face human interaction: the sight of the other person, and the sound of his or her voice. A kind face, a firm yet gentle voice, an ability to listen to the hidden meanings beyond the words and to articulate what the patient can find no words for—these are all part of the "holding" environment of therapy sessions, in which the patient should feel touched, welcomed, and safer than before. Ideally, every patient should leave each therapy session (whether group or individual) with a sense of having been "touched" in some nonphysical way that reassures even when it is also experienced as frightening.

JEAN

Apparently I succeeded in this regard early in my career with a patient named Jean, though largely for the wrong reasons. When I was still a young, idealistic social worker who believed that perseverance and good will ought to save the world, I worked in a public health clinic for children. A usually calm pediatrician sounded alarmed one day when he buzzed my office and urged me to see Jean and her 2-year-old son, Mitchell, immediately.

Mitchell was well dressed, bright-eyed, cute, and physically healthy. Jean, age 28, looked 45 and deeply troubled. She was unkempt in appearance, walked unsteadily, had scaly protuberances on her face and arms, and had a look of deep sadness in her eyes. Several missing teeth had been replaced with pieces of metal in some crude attempt at dentistry. Her messy hair and frightened demeanor gave her a wild appearance. She smiled in a somewhat contorted way, and it was clear from the first moment that she was working very hard to be present and to be socially appropriate.

Her interaction with her child was firm, loving, and sensitive to his needs, in marked contrast to what one might expect from her appearance. As she became less frightened of me in my position of authority, her eyes darted less, and she studied me carefully; eventually, she accepted my invitation to tell me about herself. Her presentation was confused and rambling at times. Occasionally she would stop talking and gaze into space. But often she made real contact with me with her eyes as she spoke sensitively about herself. The story that emerged touched me deeply—too deeply, since I must have overidentified with her from the beginning.

I no longer remember the details of her very troubled origins, but she had spent most of her adolescence and young adulthood in a state hospital. She cried about her family members, who had not wanted her, and recalled various social workers and nurses she had known over the years. She also spoke about a strange but meaningful relationship she had developed with a male patient who was much older. Reluctantly, she had agreed to have sex with him under a stairwell, although she had been terrified. During her pregnancy, contact with him was prohibited; after Mitchell was born, she was discharged from the hospital with her infant. Her heavy doses of medication were supposedly regulated during her 10-minute, monthly visits to a psychiatrist. She said that her skin condition was a reaction to her many years on psychotropic drugs.

Jean and Mitchell became one of the families I followed on a long-term basis, and I saw them in the clinic or made a home visit every week or two. I and other clinic staff members were amazed at Mitchell's relatively healthy development and the quality of mothering he seemed to receive from this strange woman. We expected serious problems to develop with the boy as he got older. Since other staff members were afraid of Jean and her odd mannerisms, they were glad to lend support to the social worker who was eager to follow her.

I also became acquainted with Jean's roommate, Sharon, who had also survived the state hospital system. She, too, had those odd metal teeth. They both welcomed me, and Jean was genuinely grateful for my presence in her life. I liked and respected Jean and she knew it. She was masterful in her ability to budget her welfare check and creative in her attempts to decorate the meager apartment I had helped her get in a housing project. She was charming in her childlike eagerness to learn about the world she had been shut out of for so long, and she seemed devoted to her son without smothering him. As she felt safer with me she was less careful in her speech, and her confusion, poor ego boundaries, and paranoia became more evident. She sometimes became annoyed when I was busy with other mothers in the clinic and was deeply hurt when I politely declined the food she wanted to cook for me. She apologized profusely for a few angry outbursts directed at me. She refused my offers to try to find a psychotherapist for her.

One day after returning from vacation, I received a desperate call from Sharon, begging me to come over. I found a trembling Jean, who tearfully told me she was determined to withdraw from the heroin her boyfriend had been giving her. Sharon had vowed to stand by her, and indeed had the loyalty to do so. I promised to help her, too, and I visited every day for a week or so until the crisis passed. My presence alone was usually comforting to Jean, but one day her body could find no peace. I recall the scene clearly: Jean was sitting on an old sofa, shaking and crying, her teeth chattering; Sharon sat on one side of her and I sat on the other, each of us holding one of her hands. Apparently I found her painful struggle intolerable, and I put my arms around her and held her. Wrapping her arms around me, she buried her head and sobbed deeply. The trembling slowly subsided, and she was moved and amazed that I was willing to hold her and to touch her "ugly" scaly skin. After that, she seemed to succeed in her withdrawal from heroin. She was thrilled with her victory and grateful to me for my help.

Several months later, I left the clinic to expand my private practice of long-term intensive psychotherapy. I wished Jean could be my patient in that setting—sick as she was, she had so much health and determination. Maybe she could really get well, I hoped, although I knew my wishes were unrealistic. Of all the people I had worked with at the clinic, it was most difficult for me to tell Jean I was leaving. She first cried and wished me well, then withdrew in hurt; she refused to say good-bye and told me I was a bad social worker. After my departure, she located my home phone number and called several times, either crying about how she missed me or threatening to hurt me, now that she knew where I lived. Nothing ever happened, and I never heard from her again. That was over 20 years ago.

Since I was not afraid of Jean's gross pathology, she took more chances with me, exposing more aspects of both her health and her illness. When she began making her threatening phone calls, I was scared, hurt, and angry. How could she treat me this way when I had been so devoted in my work with her? Certain by then that I had done everything wrong, I was too embarrassed to seek the counsel of friends, attorneys, or more experienced therapists. I just heaved a sigh of relief when the phone calls finally ceased.

Jean's behavior makes excellent sense to me now. Her severe ego boundary deficits and concomitant body image distortions are clearly evident. So are her lack of adequate mothering and fathering, and the resulting panic and inner turmoil she experienced most of the time. It is obvious now why she was tremendously confused about herself as a person and as a woman. She was a survivor; her health allowed her to function outside the hospital (a near miracle), and, beyond that, to cling to me and trust me in spite of all her previous experiences. I encouraged her to lean on me as a precondition for treating her illness. But at that time I did not understand well enough the infantile yearnings I was inadvertently stimulating.

My holding Jean physically only further thickened her unworkable transferential involvement with me. It was unworkable for three reasons:

1. I was not experienced enough then and did not understand how to work with such primitive and powerful infantile wishes for mothering.
2. The setting was not right for such work, even if I had known what to do.
3. Jean probably did not have enough emotional health to sustain

the emotional turmoil that is an unavoidable by-product of such surgery-like interventions.

Remembering Jean and learning from my errors with her have helped me, however, with other patients in settings more conducive to working through such early damage. We are all Jeans in one sense, even though many of us have been less damaged in our psychological development and our life experiences have been more fortunate. Even 20-plus years ago, I knew that people could not move beyond themselves and their character limitations without being touched on a level much deeper than that of the rational brain. I did not then understand the power of such involvement, but Jean's legacy is my continuing search for better ways of using myself to help others like her out of the emotional prisons in which they live.

NANCY (AND LAURA)

I became acquainted with Nancy several years after my final encounters with Jean. By then, I was working with several other therapists in a private practice where all our patients had regular, alternating individual and group sessions. Each patient also had the advantage of being involved with multiple therapists—both their primary individual therapist and additional cotherapists in the group. (We routinely conduct our groups with cotherapy teams of two or more therapists.)

Nancy's mother had had such serious difficulties with female identification that she had been unable to like even her own daughter. As a result, Nancy felt unwanted both as a person and as a girl; she was plagued by a deep sense of shame about her longings for closeness. In an attempt to compensate for her terrible sense of inadequacy, she developed a "tough guy" front. Her demeanor and mannerisms were not so much masculine as they were demonstrably antifeminine. Her voice was usually sharp or rough, her gestures broad and often awkward, her wit tinged with sarcasm, her laugh too loud. Not only had her attempts at softness and sensitivity been ridiculed by her mother, but they were also crudely put down by her older brothers. Her father, the only person who seemed to have had some understanding of the little girl's difficulty, was too frightened and unsteady himself to defend her against the continued harassment of the other family members.

In her work Nancy was competent and professional, often even innovative. But her personal life was lonely; her relationships with both men and women were only marginal and usually disappointing. She lived alone, literally and figuratively. Although she had eventually discovered that sexual contacts with women were more satisfying than those with men, she had given up on those, too. No relationship was ever lasting or really satisfying and meaningful to her. When Nancy's loneliness became unbearable, she sought therapy.

I was a cotherapist in Nancy's group, but since she had experienced her father as the best "mother" she had known, we therapists had concluded that it would be easier for her to become involved with a male individual therapist. Often disappointed in him and in her group, as she was with people in general, she slowly took more chances over the course of a few years and very hesitantly let her guard down. Her softness and sensitivity eventually began to show for brief moments in sessions before she would get frightened and close up again. Then, a few minutes or a few sessions later, she would feel safe enough to venture out once more. She began to lose weight and to dress in a more feminine manner, at first claiming that she was doing this just to get the therapists "off my back." But slowly she began to derive more and more pleasure from being a woman.

I became her individual therapist then. We believed that she was ready to face yet another layer of her deep fears by testing the waters of a trusting involvement with someone who could more readily evoke her painful experiences with her mother. These were often stormy times. Her previously hidden and suppressed rage was now out in the open. She hated the woman who had mothered her so poorly; consequently, she hated all other women, including me and herself. For weeks at a time, I could do nothing right. If in sessions I spoke little, I was tight and ungiving like her mother. If I intervened more frequently, I talked too much and wanted the session to go my way. "Just like my mother," she would bitterly complain, "you're not making enough room for me."

Her longings to be seen, held, nurtured, and mothered were also very powerful, however, and she sometimes feared being overwhelmed by them. It was then that I decided to have her use my couch in individual sessions, hoping that lying on this extension of me—my couch—would provide her with the sense of being "held" and help her feel safer and less threatened by her primitive fears. It did not work. Session after session, she was very tense and often silent. It was not possible for me to reach into that silence in a way she could tolerate.

One day as Nancy lay on the couch, her breathing shallow in a semiconscious attempt to choke back both her fear and her wishes for closeness and contact, I had a fantasy of physically offering her my hand. I did not then approve of ever making such a gesture in individual sessions, since I believed that the potential for confusing the patient was too great. As I observed her and her clearly evident pain, I wondered about myself and my unusual fantasy. Was I trying too hard? Was I overidentifying again? Was I confused as I had been with Jean? My intentions were obviously good, but good intentions are never a guarantee that an intervention is correct or necessary. I could find no particular anxiety within me—just compassion for Nancy, who was fighting so heroically to escape the inevitable pain brought about by her troubled background. I finally decided to take a chance and offered her my hand.

Nancy refused it, of course. And she criticized me for yet another inept attempt to help her. But I persisted in my offer, without pushing. Slowly her body began to respond. It showed in small muscular twitches in her hands, arms, and neck, and in a perceptible change in her facial expression. Her hand reached toward mine several times, each time pulling back before we touched. Her arm then began to shake. Feeling a rush of shame, as if she were doing something terribly wrong, she turned her face and then her whole body away from me, gasping in horror.

I wanted to reach for the frightened child I saw before me. It was so clear that the woman's body was only the casing that held a needy and terrified little girl. I wished to take her in my arms as I had done with Jean so many years earlier and let the warmth and steadiness of my body reassure hers. But I did not do it, having learned my lesson well. Instead I used my voice to touch her, to remind her of the reality of our situation, to coax her to turn back and not to turn away again. Once more I offered her my hand. Slowly, painfully, shivering and whimpering, she turned back. At my suggestion, she looked at me and slowly took my hand. Her bodily resistance then gave way, and she trembled, heaved, and sobbed deeply, holding on tightly to my hand. On her own, she added her other hand, cradling mine in both of hers.

A few minutes before the end of the session, I gently withdrew my hand from Nancy's and encouraged her to reflect on what had happened in her and to her in this unusually powerful hour. It was almost impossible for her to think then; her feelings were still so strong. So I asked her to sit up and focus on me. With her feet on the floor and her eyes observing the real me, her therapist in the present time frame, she could eventually speak sensitively about the painful longings of the child inside her. She had always tried hard to hide these yearnings for a good mother because they seemed shameful to her.

By the following year, Nancy felt safe enough in her group to expose and experience her hurt openly sometimes. She spoke with difficulty in one session about my apparent insensitivity to her and my not seeming to understand the depth of her pain. My cotherapist helped her talk directly to me about loving me and wanting more from me—an understandably difficult task for this patient especially. His sensitivity and calm, firm, male voice were very reassuring to her and gave her enough support to proceed. As she spoke tearfully and haltingly, her right shoulder tightened visibly. He helped her tell me about the painful tension, and persistently encouraged her to ask me to "Rub it, please." Conquering her shame again and again, and tempted to withdraw with every breath, she pressed forward, never giving in to her enormous fear.

As always, I asked for permission to touch her even though she had requested it. And she again cringed as she granted it. She understood that the physical intervention had nothing to do with either rubbing or massaging a tight muscle. It would instead be a further step toward facing the irrational fears that dominated her body. I stood behind her, one hand on her painful shoulder, the other on her forehead. The back of her head rested against my abdomen. Reminded to breathe deeply through an open mouth, she began to shake and cry, visibly fighting her tendency to hide her face in shame. At my suggestion, she held on to my arm with both hands as she continued to sob and whimper alternately. This lasted for several minutes. A few group members spoke about their reactions to what Nancy was going through; some were envious, others frightened.

"Well, I'm hurt! You never touch me that way," Laura whined in my direction. Her face quickly took on the pouty look of a hurt 4-year-old, and her toes turned inward toward each other without her realizing it, as a little girl's feet might do in their patent leather Mary Janes. "It's obvious that you don't like me as much as Nancy. You just put up with me because I pay you." She folded her arms, raised her chin slightly, and averted her gaze, really sounding like a little girl.

Nancy's freedom to regress temporarily without being ridiculed and without suffering any actual damage enabled the otherwise controlled Laura to do the same. It was a safe setting, indeed. The visible, beneficial effects of the work with Nancy had made it possible for others, too, to repress less. Residues of very old hurt were bubbling up.

Laura had been infantilized and overindulged by both parents. They experienced her as a "blessing" bestowed on them late in life. Although now a young adult, she was crippled by her infantile expectations that the world would always provide for her. This was not the first time she had appeared to be like a 4-year-old, but these character habits had never before been so obvious or so openly observable. Laura was often on the verge of leaving therapy when pushed to take more and more responsibility for herself. At our insistence, she was now paying for half her therapy on her own rather than depending on her parents—a major achievement for Laura, but one about which she still needed to complain frequently.

Laura was right about my never touching her the way I had Nancy. It would clearly have been the wrong message, at least at this point of her therapy, and would have confused her. As a baby and toddler, she had been physically held, cuddled, and attended to too much by her anxious mother, who was trying to allay her own anxiety. Even now the mother occasionally addressed Laura in baby talk. Instead of touching Laura or allowing her to withdraw after her tantrum, I insisted that she straighten her feet and adjust her face in spite of the storm of feelings that had just passed through her, and that she talk thoughtfully about what she had experienced. It took a great deal of effort on her part, but finally she spoke sadly about the little girl who had never received the firm pressure she needed to grow up to be a competent adult. The contrast with Nancy was now obvious even to Laura: Nancy had learned to behave like a competent adult while still a child, since in her family there was no room for the little girl. Later on, after I had returned to my seat and several other patients had spoken about themselves, Nancy reflected easily on her current calm and pain-free state, contrasting it with her tight, contorted body and powerful feelings of just a few minutes earlier. In so doing, she began to integrate another therapeutic experience—another small step in the corrective emotional work she was engaged in.

"Even though we have no conscious memory of our early experiences, our body remembers. We adapt to them or perish," says Bar-Levav (1988, p. 323). Wilhelm Reich (1942) recognized many years ago that the "muscular armor" is formed in response to subjectively fear-filled experiences during the period of character formation. Considerable work has also been done in the past 25 years by Alexander Lowen (1975), Charles Kelley (1974, 1988, 1993) and many others (e.g., Durkin, Glatzer, Munzer, O'Hearne, & Spotnitz, 1972) to expand our understanding of these concepts and to enhance our ability to work with the body directly. Strange as it may still sound to some, it is clear now that muscles like those in Nancy's shoulder are indeed the seat of "memories." Somehow that area of the body became Nancy's locus for storing fear and other forms of emotional pain. We do not yet know the exact mechanisms of how or why one region rather than another is "chosen" for this purpose, but our recognition of the existence of physiological memory traces allows us to address the musculature directly. An intervention that temporarily loosens the level of tension in a burdened shoulder, for example, converts the physical pressure into affects and makes room for experiencing feelings as such and for vocally expressing long-buried fear, rage, or hurt. When this occurs in a group session, the presence of others who are not critical undercuts the patient's lifelong sense of shame associated with the open expression of feelings. The "certainty" that strong feelings can be safely experienced only in private and in hiding eventually gives way. Consequently, it was reasonable to expect that the general level of anxiety in Nancy's body would subside as the shoulder, like her vocal cords and other muscle groups, no longer bore the extra pressure.

Patients sometimes begin to believe that the therapist's touch (as well as other well-timed therapeutic interventions) has magical powers. This sense ought to be quickly and repeatedly defused. Otherwise the way is open to a positive transference "cure," which is transitory and unreal and can never heal emotional illness. The power of physical touch is great, since the body (and "soul") long for the exquisite sensitivity of a perfect "mother" in whose literal or figurative arms one feels safe. Patients must have such experiences with their therapists in order to elicit formerly frozen affects that block healthy functioning of body parts (including the ability of the cortex to reason under continual pressure), but the observing ego must always put each such experience in perspective without a long delay (Bar-Levav, 1988, p. 225). Eventually patients learn to mother themselves, and then they neither cling to others nor shrink away from intimate contact.

DARREN

Patients with an "as-if" defensive structure are often experienced by psychotherapists as being among the most difficult to treat. Specific forms of physical touch can be useful to some of these patients, but the circumstances in which such interventions are utilized must be very clearly delineated. Terrified at the core, such patients protect themselves against perceived emotional dangers by adapting to what they believe is pleasing to others. Emotionally they resemble chameleons, with many shades of color available to them to camouflage themselves in order to seek a sense of safety. This adaptive process takes place automatically on an unconscious level whenever danger is perceived; consequently, such individuals are unaware of its presence. Such patients do not mean to fool their therapists or others, since they themselves are blind to their "as-if" changes. Although they manage to keep their massive anxiety in check, such patients have an unclear sense of who they really are.

Darren, a middle-aged psychotherapist, is such a person. Now, in the middle phase of his own therapy, enough cracks in his defensive walls have been produced that he can no longer deny his nearly overwhelming tendency to try to please others, particularly women. Born into a large family with other siblings before and after him, he understandably developed this way of being in the hope that he would be better seen and perhaps even praised. He became a rigidly efficient man who, though well liked, condemned himself to walk a narrow path that always demanded near-perfection. Any slip on his part, any deviation, led to anxiety, self-deprecation, and self-reproach. Darren's apparent "giving" to others was a facade behind which he hid his desperate wish to "be given," as well as his harsh treatment of himself. His need to "give" overdetermined his choice of profession and the quality of his relationships, but it did not save him from living with debilitating anxiety. This finally pushed him to seek therapy.

Darren's ready smile and compulsive helpfulness were barriers to his experiencing his rage or panic in the group. At the suggestion of his therapists, he agreed not to help any of his fellow group members in any way for 3 months. At first, he used to chuckle as he caught himself again and again reaching for a box of tissues, eagerly offering it to someone who was crying. He eventually began to grip the arms of his chair and to grit his teeth to force himself not to make helpful gestures and interpretations. Finally he could tolerate it no longer. Deeply buried anger and impatience bubbled up in sessions as he complained openly and powerfully about the "stupid" suggestion of his therapists. Eventually he even found some characteristics of his fellow group members to be annoying, and he said so openly. His anger frightened him. Without his compulsive "niceness" to help hide his rage, his body now tended to tighten and to rigidify. The fear of rejection resulting from his open expressions of anger then combined with his fear of losing control and of becoming violent, and all his feelings again went "underground." Temporary numbness and a flat- tened affect sometimes followed such breakthroughs—a not uncommon sequence in patients reaching this point.

Physical touching can be most helpful at such times. With patients like Darren, the sense of being exposed and therefore grossly unsafe is so great that the tendency to re-repress the emerging affects becomes nearly overwhelming. The sight of the therapist and the sound of his or her voice are often no longer enough to "hold" such a patient in the here and now, since the powerful "new" affects appear subjectively as a threat to the integrity of the less than fully competent ego boundaries. A firm and prolonged physical touch on the arms, back, shoulders, forehead, and/or neck can often literally "remind" the patient's body that the current situation is, in reality, safe. The terror- filled body is thus reassured that even the strongest feelings that temporarily cloud the brain and confuse the observing ego are not in fact dangerous.

This, indeed, was what happened to Darren over and over again.

One of the male therapists would firmly press his hands on Darren's shoulders or support his forehead with one hand and the back of his head with the other, while insisting that he keep his mouth and eyes open and breathe deeply. Darren would again and again thus regain enough of his sense of equilibrium that he could continue to experience and to openly express his previously hidden terrible fear. This was often associated with deep sobbing. The little boy who always felt constrained to be sweet and helpful, and who had to choke back all traces of his hurt and powerful rage, was now free and able to feel it all as such. Such experiences slowly release the pressure that has been locked in the body for a lifetime. The deep crying is always followed by a sense of profound relief.

The touch of a male therapist's hand at such times is usually more effective than that of a female, particularly with a male patient. The unconscious wish at such moments of daring to reexperience old and long-buried subjective horrors is to melt into the softness of a woman, exactly as a frightened baby would burrow into its mother's bosom. But the immediate need of a patient like Darren (whether male or female) is to reestablish the sense of boundaries and separateness, ideally almost in the midst of such a "regressive" progression. Thus, a physically firm masculine touch is usually the medium of choice.

MARJORIE

One of the major goals of psychotherapy ought to be the development of the ability to self-mother. This is an essential capacity for healthy adult living (Bar-Levav, 1988, p. 329). Without it, people must always look to others for nurturance. Proper attention to one's body and to its real needs is one important function of self-mothering. Another is properly satisfying one's own real emotional needs, which can and must be distinguished from indulging one's infantile wishes. Those who have been inadequately mothered as infants and as small children hardly ever develop this ability for loving self-care, and proper therapy must therefore include work in this neglected and underdeveloped area of the personality.

The case of Marjorie is a good example of this. The poor mothering this 24-year-old had received was evident from her appearance. Seriously overweight, she walked with an awkward gait and always appeared unkempt. No matter how hard she tried—and she made great efforts—she was unable to pull herself together completely. If her clothes were clean and pressed, she had runs in her hose. If her makeup was attractive and appropriate, her hair was a mess. If her skirt was the right length, her shoes were scuffed or showed outright wear and tear. She usually looked like a young child in need of help in dressing herself. She was often embarrassed about her appearance and deeply ashamed of her inability to do everything right. Bright and competent, Marjorie did well in her graduate studies, but she spent an enormous amount of time in silent ruminative deliberations involving self-blame.

In individual sessions, Marjorie's body eventually felt "safe" enough to relax some of its chronic tension. Then she would sadly cry for herself or talk thoughtfully, freed for a few minutes from her almost continual self-recriminations. But in the group this was more difficult. There she was more frightened by the multiple stimuli and usually felt a need to be on guard. Although able to be sensitive and helpful to other group members, talking about herself led quickly to ruminative struggles to be "perfect." This was followed by a deep sense of shame when she felt she had failed again.

Marjorie was hurt, embarrassed, and certain that I was making fun of her the first time I suggested she sit on my lap in a group session. At my urging she talked about these feelings rather than withdrawing. Encouraged by her peers to try out what seemed to be a very strange suggestion, she anxiously and very slowly joined me, trying hard to support some of her own weight for fear that it would injure me. (I have found that my lap can in fact tolerate quite a bit of weight for a few minutes, and that usually only a few minutes are needed for a Marjorie to take one or two new steps away from the physiological prison of her body.)

At first Marjorie's body was jumpy and tense, and she was driven to ruminate about returning to her seat. It was enough now, she said, and I really should remember to work with some of the other patients who also needed my help. Firmly placing both my hands on her shoulders and back, I invited her to look at one of the other group members and describe her experience. Her quivering body began to settle down as she spoke about how surprised she was at being comfortable and feeling somewhat comforted. This did not last for long. Soon she was driven again by her rising anxiety to ruminate about liking all this too much, and to try to convince me that she ought to go back to her seat. The continued physical reassurance, combined with my observations that the little girl inside her grown body was probably unaccustomed to being held in a safe lap, helped her slow down. She began to talk sadly and thoughtfully, with specific examples, about the child who was always afraid to ask for much and who was always on guard against Mother's unpredictable outbursts and Father's demands for perfection. I asked if that child knew any songs. Bouncing her slightly on my knee, I joined her in singing "Row, Row, Row Your

Boat"; she then continued singing on her own, giggling like a little girl who was no longer self-conscious.

Marjorie did not even want to intellectualize about what this all meant, and I would have discouraged her from doing so. She simply and innocently enjoyed her own laughter, "mothering" herself once the little girl inside her had absorbed my steadiness. When space is made for the legitimate needs of the frightened child, more room exists for the adult. This, indeed, was how Marjorie walked back to her seat. She was less awkward, although only temporarily. Physical touch is not a character-altering magic, and the body overcomes its familiar ways only very gradually.

Following such episodes, patients generally experience real freedom from their normally high level of anxiety—at least for a few minutes, sometimes a little longer. During such periods, not only is the body generally more relaxed, but the characteristic facial expression usually also changes. As the tension level of all muscles is temporarily lessened, vision and hearing often become more acute, and gait and other movements may become smoother. Hundreds of similar experiences are needed in a full course of successful psychotherapy, during which the physiology changes in basic ways and the patient's body slowly sheds the suit of armor it has "worn" for years. Eventually, a much more relaxed state of being becomes the rule rather than the exception. This is a necessary part of overcoming chronic anxiety and depression.

GUIDELINES FOR THE USE OF PHYSICAL TOUCH

Physical contact with patients is often a necessary tool in intensive therapy that aims at healing emotional illness and not merely relieving symptoms. But such a powerful tool should be used judiciously, only under very specific conditions that protect the patient from abuse and also guard the therapist. Physical touch can confuse therapists whose ego boundaries are not well delineated, which is why clear ground rules are necessary. The potential for abuse in utilizing these powerful techniques is great, even with the best of intentions.

The following guidelines ought to be carefully observed at all times:

1. *Beginning therapists should never touch their patients under any circumstances.* At best, they will confuse them slightly; at worst, they will open the door to distortions that can put them in real danger, as I did with Jean. Only experienced therapists should use physical techniques,

and they should do so only after they have mastered other "holding" techniques and have a clear understanding of physiological memory.

2. *A real adult relationship between patient and therapist must clearly exist.* This serves as a solid foundation for clarification of any transferential distortions, especially those that might be stimulated by physical touch. Clear arrangements regarding time and money clarify the purpose of the relationship. Not only hugs but even routine handshakes are best avoided in intensive psychotherapy, to emphasize the basic difference in nature between this relationship and a social one. Bar-Levav (1988) comments:

> In a sense, two parallel relationships must develop and remain in existence between therapist and patient—a real one and a therapeutic one. The basis of the real relationship is complete honesty and mutual respect, combined with a two-sided commitment to remain involved even in the presence of powerful expressions of hurt, anger, or irrational fear by the patient. (Therapists are expected to be essentially free of these, at least in relation to their patients.) But in the therapeutic relationship room is made for the expression of any thoughts and all of the patient's feelings, without limiting their intensity and with no need to hold back or hide anything. What is unpleasant, painful, or embarrassing to the patient finds room here, and so does any criticism, disappointment, and anger at the therapist. (p. 222)

> The therapeutic relationship is often extremely stormy, but as long as it occurs within a real-relationship that holds the patient lovingly, firmly, and consistently, all the storms eventually subside. (p. 236)

3. *Physical touch of any kind is contraindicated at the beginning of therapy,* in order to help establish the real relationship on a firm footing. At the beginning of therapy, patients' involvement is almost always based largely on positive transference. At the very least, physical touch at that time is likely to overload the holding capacity of the real relationship. At worst, it may damage the patient by causing him or her to leave therapy or to develop a psychotic transference.

4. *The therapist must be ready, willing, and able to make a long-term commitment to the patient and the therapy process.* Any and all feelings stimulated by physical touch must be worked through; this may well require working through the most basic developmental defects in the character structure. Touching physiological memories and attempting to alter habitual pathways of physiological response constitute a difficult and lengthy process that should never be undertaken lightly. Since the therapist's major tool is his or her self, the therapist ought to be present throughout the entire process.

5. *A clear contract that separates actions and feelings must already be in effect in the relationship between the patient and the therapist, and among all the patients in a group.* No action, especially physical touching, is ever permitted by either patient or therapist without requesting and obtaining explicit verbal permission in every case anew. Since feelings often masquerade as thoughts, it is essential to double- and triple-check the rational basis of any wish to act in any form (Bar-Levav, 1993a). It must be remembered that physical touching can merely be a way to discharge feelings, and thus can impede the therapeutic work.

6. *Physical touching is safest for patient and therapist alike if done almost exclusively in a group setting, and hardly ever in individual sessions.* This serves to protect patients from possible abuse by emotionally immature therapists, and to protect therapists from distortions by patients that could lead to lawsuits. Patients need to have both group and individual sessions that take place on a regular basis. The processing and integration of experiences involving physical touch are most usefully done in the presence of peers, who serve as very effective reminders of current reality.

7. *Ideally, a cotherapist should be present whenever physical touch is applied.* The reasoning here is the same as that of a male gynecologist who routinely has a female nurse present when performing a pelvic examination. The additional importance of such a practice is self-evident in the age of so-called "recovered" early memories of abuse. Furthermore, the cotherapist may see indications or contraindications to which a colleague is insensitive. Together they can decide which of them is more suited to the patient's needs at the moment, in terms of gender and possible transference reactions (Torraco, 1995, p. 24).

8. *Before physical touching is used, its value should be weighed in comparison with all other possibilities.* Touch is only one of many possible interventions an experienced therapist has at his or her disposal at any one moment. The ongoing work of intensive psychotherapy requires an ability to be emotionally open, involved, and available, based on reasonably intact and flexible ego boundaries. Such demanding requirements develop only with emotional maturity and time, and they are unlike the demands of other learned professions. "The work itself exposes us and makes us vulnerable to experiencing any and all feelings with the greatest intensity" (Bar-Levav, 1993b, p. 14). Consequently, therapists must check and recheck themselves to guard against possible lapses in judgment caused by strong feelings. Since all people harbor yearnings to be touched and held, even an experienced therapist can momentarily overidentify with a patient and touch him or her at the wrong time and for the wrong reason.

9. *Touching should only be used to move a patient through and beyond*

a layer of fear that "freezes" his or her ability to benefit from other interventions. Fear can paralyze the physiology, the feelings, and/or the thinking, and can thus cause the patient either not to move forward or to regress. Physical touch is one of several possible avenues of intervention at such times. Touching must never be used to gratify infantile wishes. It is *never* indicated because it "feels good" to either patient or therapist, or because the therapist does not know what else to do.

10. *Sexually suggestive or stimulating touch must always be avoided; even an arm or shoulder can never be fondled.* Therapists not only must avoid the genitals, but must take extra care even when touching the chest or abdomen. Experienced therapists are likely to be neutralized themselves to zones of potential confusion, but patients can easily become confused without knowing it when they are emotionally very open and therefore more vulnerable. Erotic transferences or psychotic-like, unworkable early preverbal transferences can develop and harden if exquisite care is not taken at crucial moments.

11. *Touch must always be firm, have a clear and easy-to-define purpose, and be relatively brief.* The patient's tissues will respond to a tentative, unsure touch; they will "know" that this touch cannot be trusted. A therapist's touch can never be a caress, and any sort of casual touch is at best useless.

Heeding these factors, we can safely touch our patients from time to time, thus expanding the variety of techniques available to us in this difficult, challenging, and exciting work. But whether or not we actually use physical touch, we hold lives in our hands no less than a surgeon facing a draped patient on the table does. We need intrusive techniques to reach insidious pieces of pathology, but they must always be used prudently and sensitively. Our patients count on us to remain vigilant that what we do is in their best interests and not our own.

REFERENCES

Bar-Levav, R. (1988). *Thinking in the shadow of feelings: A new understanding of the hidden forces that shape individuals and societies.* New York: Simon & Schuster.

Bar-Levav, R. (1993a). A rationale for physical touching in psychotherapy. *International Journal of Psychotherapy and Critical Thought, 1*(1), 5–7.

Bar-Levav, R. (1993b). A real case of near fatal attraction. *Voices, 29,* 10–14.

Durkin, H. E., Glatzer, H. T., Munzer, J., O'Hearne, J. J., & Spotnitz, H. (1972). To touch or not to touch. *International Journal of Group Psychotherapy, 22,* 444–469.

Kelley, C. R. (1974). *Education in feeling and purpose* (rev. ed.). Vancouver, WA: Kelley/Radix.

Kelley, C. R. (1988). *Body contact in radix work.* Vancouver, WA: Kelley/Radix.

Kelley, C. R. (1993). Touching in radix work. *International Journal of Psychotherapy and Critical Thought, 1*(1), 21–23.

Lowen, A. (1975). *Bioenergetics.* New York: Coward, McCann & Geoghegan.

Reich, W. (1942). *The function of the orgasm.* New York: Orgone Institute Press.

Torraco, P. (1995). Rage without violence. *Voices, 31,* 16–25.

INDEX